3. NIX-KUNER

Foot Point-Zone Massage Therapy

Written by   Shan Renying
                 Yu Meng'ai
Revised by   Wang Guocai
Translated by   Lu Yubin
                  Wang Yan
                  Ma Xinyuan

Shandong Science and Technology Press

First Edition 1997
ISBN 7−5331−1891−X

Foot Point-Zone Massage Therapy

Written	by	Shan Renying
		Yu Meng'ai
Revised	by	Wang Guocai
Translated	by	Lu Yubin, Wang Yan
		Ma Xinyuan
Editor in charge		Ma Wannian

Published by Shandong Science and Technology Press
16 Yuhan Road, 250002, Jinan, China
Printed by Shandong Binzhou Xinhua Printing House
Distributed by China International Book Trading Corporation
35 Chegongzhuang Xilu, Beijing 100044, China
P. O. Box 399, Beijing, China
Printed in the People's Republic of China

Preface

Foot Point-Zone Massage Therapy is one volume of *The Series of Traditional Chinese Medicine for Foreign Readers*.

This book is designed and written for foreign TCM practitioners and patients who hope that they can apply this therapy in their clinical practice or treat their diseases and keep their fit by themselves.

Foot massage therapy is a traditional therapy in China. Different from the foot massage therapy in other countries, this therapy in TCM is based on both the theories of TCM and the achievements of modern science. Therefore, it is more valuable and practical in the clinic.

This book contains three major parts. Part one is a general introduction to the concept of foot point-zone massage therapy; part two involves the commonly used points and reflecting areas with a detailed description of their locations, manipulations and indications; and part three deals with application of this therapy in treatment of various kinds of diseases, in which a general description of the diseases, essentials of diagnosis, massage treatment of the disease and remarks on the treatment are made.

This book can be used as both a textbook for foreign TCM learners and the foreign TCM practitioners. In addition, it may also be adopted as a reference book for Western doctors who hope have some knowledge of TCM.

Compiler

Contents

General Introduction ··· 1
  1. Foot—the indicator of the health ··················· 1
  2. Foot—a key to open the door of health and longevity ··· 4
  3. Brief introduction to the foot point-zone massage therapy ··· 5

Basic Knowledge of Foot Point-Zone Massage Therapy ··· 7
  1. Effect of the foot point-zone massage ············· 7
    (1) Promoting blood circulation by moving blood and removing blood stasis ···················· 7
    (2) Relieving fatigue and enhancing the resistant ability of the body against diseases ············ 8
    (3) Treating inflammation, arresting pain and promoting tissues repairement ················ 8
    (4) Promoting flow of Qi and Blood to regulate functional balance of organs ···················· 8
    (5) Regulating the whole body comprehensively ··· 9
  2. Principles for massage on point-zone in feet ·· 9
  3. Advantages of massage on point-zone of foot ·· 10
    (1) Wide indications ······································· 10
    (2) Reliable and safe without any side or toxic effects ·· 10
    (3) Diagnosing disease early and treating diseases quickly ·· 10
    (4) Simple and easy to perform, spread and popularize ·· 11

    (5) Cultivating one's moral, enhancing therapeutic
        effects and preserving one's health ············ 11
4. Commonly used manipulations in foot point-
   zone massage ·································· 11
5. The reducing and reinforcing effects of the
   manipulations ································· 19
6. Commonly used instruments and techniques in
   the foot point-zone massage ····················· 19
    (1) Massage with massage rod ················ 20
    (2) Treading on glass balls with barefoot ········ 20
    (3) Stepping a bamboo rod ···················· 20
    (4) Stepping the crossbean of a stool ············ 20
7. Attentions for foot point-zone massage ············ 20
8. Restraint for foot point-zone massage ············ 21

Structure and Function of Foot, Important Points and Reflecting Zones ································· 23

1. Structure and function of foot ····················· 23
2. Channels of foot ································ 25
    (1) The Stomach Channel of
        Foot-Yangming ··························· 25
    (2) The Gallbladder Channel of
        Foot-Shaoyang ··························· 25
    (3) The Bladder Channel of Foot-Taiyang ······ 25
    (4) The Spleen Channel of Foot-Taiyin ············ 25
    (5) The Liver Channel of Foot-Jueyin ············ 26
    (6) The Kidney Channel of Foot-Shaoyin ········ 26
3. Important points in foot ························· 29
    (1) Important points of the Stomach Channel of
        Foot-Yangming ··························· 29
    (2) Important points of the Bladder Channel of
        Foot-Taiyang ····························· 31
    (3) Important points of the Gallbladder Channel
        of Foot-Shaoyang ························· 34
    (4) Important points of the Kidney Channel of
        Foot-Shaoyin ····························· 37

     (5) Important points of the Liver Channel of Foot-Jueyin 39
     (6) Important points of the Spleen Channel of Foot-Taiyin 41
     (7) Extra and special points in the foot region 44
  4. The reflecting zones of foot 46
     (1) The reflecting zones of the right foot 47
     (2) The reflecting zones of the left foot 47
     (3) The reflecting zones of the lateral side of foot 47
     (4) The reflecting zones of the medial side of foot 47
     (5) The reflecting zones on the dorsum of foot 47
  5. Brief introduction to each of the reflecting zones 53
     (1) The reflecting zones of the right sole 53
     (2) The reflecting zones of the left sole 60
     (3) The reflecting zones in the lateral side of foot 61
     (4) The reflecting zones in the medial side of foot 63
     (5) The reflecting zones on the dorsum of foot 65

Treatment of Diseases with Foot Point-Zone Massage Therapy 68
  Diseases of the Internal Medicine 68
  Surgical Diseases 127
  Pediatric Diseases 140
  Gynecological Diseases 143
  Diseases of the Mouth, Ears, Eyes and Nose 155
  Dermatological Diseases 167

General Introduction

*E*ach part of the human body contains the information of the whole body. Looking at the sole of the human body, you will find the different reflecting zones of the different parts of the human body, which are distributed in the same way as the different component parts of the human body. What doesn't this mean? what will happen to these zones or points? and what can we do with these zones or points?

1. Foot—the indicator of the health

Each foot of a person consists of 26 bones, of which 7 are tarsal bones, 5 are ankle bones, and 14 are phalanges. These bones are connected with each other by the muscles, ligaments and fiber bundles in order to meet the needs of the functional activities of the foot. Numerous nerve branches, nerve endings and various kinds of internal and external sensors are distributed over the foot and blood circulation in the foot is plentiful. These sensors response to stimuli quickly and can send back the information to the brain promptly, so they can do different judgements and receive instructions to regulate their own states and meet the requirements of different environments. The foot, located in the lowest position of the human body, is the farest from the heart, so speed of blood flow in the foot is the slowest. The acid metabolic products, the calcium not utilised and the other metal ions as well as the macromolecular organic substances in the blood, due to long-standing vertical movements of the human body and the effect of attraction of the gravitation, are prone to sink at the bottom of the foot, and will irritate related reflecting zones to produce vicious stimuli to the corresponding organs and cause functional disturbance of the organs if the sediment lasts a long time, especially in the case of being ill with some diseases or presentation of atherosclerosis in the middle aged or the aged. These pathological products, then, will form small hard masses or streak-like nodules in the reflecting zones they stay, which, as a kind of pathologic hard nodular tissues existing in the reflecting zones, will further stimulate their related organs and the functional activities of the organs constantly, leading to organic diseases of the organs. From this it can be seen that the structure and functional state of the foot tissues have a direct influence on the health of the whole body, so the foot is called "the second heart of the human body".

Clinically, the above mentioned pathologic hard nodular tissues are termed positive responding substances. Because most patients will present pain when these nodular or streak-like hard mass tissues are pressed, they are also called painful tendinous nodules or painful tendinous streak. So, diseases can be diagnosed by palpating the reflecting zones or the foot points, since existence of positive reflecting points on the foot suggests pathological changes of the related organs or functional systems. Besides, direct massage with different manipulations can be carried out on the foot points or zones presenting the positive responding substances to soften, smash or grind the hard nodules. What is more, the manipulations can improve the blood circulation in the foot reflexibly, accelerate blood flow and clear away the pathologic or toxic substances accumulating in the local zones. This will further improve the blood flow throughout the whole body and help the diseased organs or functional systems to restore to normal gradually by eliminating the stimuli lesion. Therefore, the foot is also described as the "third eye of the human body", which means that various kinds of factors influencing the health including the senility, diseases, functional states of the

Zang-Fu organs and disharmony of Yin and Yang, can be detected by means of the conditions of the foot reflecting zones or points.

As early as 2000 years before, our ancestors had adopted the foot point massage therapy. In *Yang Shen Fang (Prescriptions for Building Up Health)*, a book unearthed in the Tombs of Mawang of Han dynasty in Changsha, Hunan Province, in 1993, it was recorded a medicated bowl made up with little cock died of sting by wasp and date paste had been applied in the foot massage to warm up Yang Qi and strengthen the strength. In the period from Warring States Period to the Qing and Han dynasties, the foot points massage therapy was further widely applied and summarized, and preliminary exploration was made on the physiology, pathology and the role of the foot in the treatment of diseases theoretically. Plentiful descriptions on this can be found in the book *Huang Di Nei Jing (The Yellow Emperor's Internal Classic)* written in this period, in which it is pointed out that the foot is closely related to the twelve regular channels, the five Zang organs, the six Fu organs and the five sense organs on the face both in structure and physiologic functions. "The foot depends on blood for its walk", so the movement, gait, hot and cold sensation and the nutritive states and lustreness of the muscles and skin of the foot can reflect whether Qi and Blood are sufficient and whether the human body is healthy. Pathologically, it is believed in this book that "When Cold and Dampness invade the human body, they attack the foot first". So, it is an important measure to take a good care of the foot and keep it warm in preventing pathogens from invading the human body. In treatment of disease, it is advocated that "Diseases on the head can be treated by treating the foot", which means that points on foot can be used to treat diseases of the whole body. For example, Yongquan and Kunlun can be selected to treat Yin Bi syndrome marked by abdominal fullness, lumbago, constipation, pain in the shoulder, back, neck and nape and occasional dizziness; and Yongquan and Yinlingquan can be selected to treat febrile diseases with sudden pain around the umbilicus and fullness in the chest and hypochondrium.

From the above we can see that foot is not only what carries us to walk, but also the indicator of our health.

2. Foot—a key to open the door to health and longevity

A proverb goes that "Foot is the first aged in the human body". So, condition of the foot is often taken as a sign of the senility of the human body. For instance, a person with presenility is often said to be "not so old, but walk like a very old person", and a healthy old man is often said to be "white hair with a boyish face and a flexible walk." It is pointed out in *Huang Di Nei Jing* (*The Yellow Emperor's Internal Classic*) that "When man is over 64 years old, he will have a heavy sensation of the body and his gait become difficult.", which means that as a result of decline of the Kidney Qi and the ensuing deficiency of the five Zang organs, a man will present heaviness of the body and unsteadiness of gait when he is 64 years old or so. Exogenous pathogens of many diseases of the human body invade the human body by attacking the foot first and will present various kinds of symptoms or signs on the foot. For example, "Numbness of foot arises from Blood stagnancy in the foot, and exuberance of Yang Qi will cause hot sensation over the soles"; "When pathogenic Dryness is prevalent, many people will have pain in the foot"; "Exuberance of Dryness may cause hotness of the foot skin"; " Stagnation of Fire will cause a warm sensation over the sole"; and "Cold foot will be exhibited in the case of Yin Qi accumulating in the lower part of the body." Therefore, it is of prime importance to take a good care of the foot in the health preservation and aging prevention of the body. Based on this understanding, therapeutic plans of foot preservation and foot treatment were, for the first time, recorded in a silk book *Mai Fa* (*Method of Taking Pulse*) unearthed in the Tomb of Mawang of Hang dynasty in Changsha, Hunan Province. It is said in this book that "Treating disease by cooling the head and warming the foot based on the principle of reducing the Excess and reinforcing the Deficiency", indicating that keeping the foot warm is very important in treatment of disease. When *Huang Di Nei Jing* (*The Yellow Emperor's Internal Classic*) mentions the health preservation theories and principles, it said that " A holy person follows changes of the heaven to nourish his head, changes of the earth to support his foot, and changes of the society to strengthen his five Zang organs. " Since the Spring-Autumn and Warring States Period, such foot health preservation therapy, foot Qigong therapy, foot sport therapy and other foot therapy as drug sticking therapy, drug-smearing therapy, drug-stamping therapy, foot fugimating therapy, hot compress therapy, acupuncture therapy, medicated bowl smearing therapy and mind-concentration therapy on the foot, which all take the foot points as the stimulation points, have come into being gradually and widely applied. For thousands of years, the clinical practice of doctors in both China and other countries have proved that man can maintain his health and keep longevity through applying various kinds of foot therapies and foot health preservation measures.

3. Brief introduction to the foot point-zone massage therapy

Foot point-zone massage therapy is a therapy to build up one's health, prevent and treat disease by applying various kinds of massage manipulations of traditional Chinese medicine to the selected important points and reflecting zones on the foot under the guidance of the meridian theory and Zang-xiang theory of TCM and the principles of physiology and pathology of Western medicine.

The important points on the foot are also called the foot points, which mainly indicate the Jing-Well points, the Ying-Spring points, the Shu-Stream points, the Jing-River points, the He-Sea points (which are collectively known as the five Shu points), the Yuan-Primary points, the Luo-Connecting points, the Xi-Cleft points, the eight confluential points, the crossing points of the three Yang channels of foot (The Stomach Channel of Foot-Yangming, the Gallbladder Channel of Foot-Shaoyang, and the Bladder Channel of Foot-Taiyang) and the three Yin channels of foot (The Spleen Channel of Foot-Taiyin, the Liver Channel of Foot Jueyin, and the Kidney Channel of Foot-Shaoyin), and the channel points, the extra points and experiential effective points which are extremely effective for some diseases. The foot reflecting zones refer to the zones listed in the surface of the foot skin and having special intrinsic connecting ways with corresponding internal organs where the nerve ends and the internal or external sensors congeal.

When a disease is to be treated with foot massage therapy, a prescription composed by the foot points and the foot reflecting zones should be formulated first according to the Syndrome identified as well as the principles of therapeutics in both Chinese and Western medicines. Then, various kinds of massage manipulations are applied to the foot points and foot reflecting zones in sequence according to the prescription. The force exerted on manipulation should be different in different patients' constitutions and illness. It may be gentle, slow and soft or deep, heavy and quick. On the one hand, these manipulations composed of various kinds of dynamic factors such as the severity, frequency and direction of the force, can penetrate into the depth of the human body along the route of "channel-viscera related" by acting on the foot points to irritate the channel Qi and induce Qi to be where the disease is. So, they can promote flow of Qi, remove Blood Stasis, dredge channels and collaterals, reinforce the Deficiency, reduce the Excess, support the Vital Qi, eliminate pathogens, regulate the function of Zang-Fu organs and harmonize Yin and Yang. On the other hand, these manipulations can excite the nerve ends and the internal or external sensors congealling in the foot reflecting zones, produce the afferent impulse which will spread to the spine nervous cells dominating the corresponding internal organs along the afferent route of the nerve reflection arc and exert influence on the functional states of the internal organs and the different systems, thus performing their therapeutic effects.

Foot point massage therapy is a product of integrity of Chinese and Western medicines. It is a combination of the traditional point massage in TCM and the massage in the light of the nerve segments in Western medicine based on the theories of both Chinese and Western medicine. The channel effect and the specific effect of the nerve reflection in the foot massage therapy supplement each other, and this therapy is of great practical value in health preservation and rehabilitating medicine.

Basic Knowledge of Foot Point-Zone Massage Therapy

*F*oot massage therapy is simple to learn and carry out, but it is necessary for one to master some basic knowledge about it such as the effects, the prinicples of application and the manipulations of this therapy as well as the commonly used tools in application of this therapy so that one can learn and apply this therapy correctly and effectively.

1. Effect of the foot point-zone massage

(1) Promoting blood circulation by moving blood and removing blood stasis

Blood stasis in TCM indicates sluggish flow of blood in mild cases and formation of congealed Blood as a pathologic product in severe cases. Stimuli produced in the foot massage can cause changes of the microcirculation in the local zone, dilate small vessels, increase filling of tissues, remove or reduce sediments, help to discharge the metabolic products out of the body as soon as possible, improve the blood circulation in the tissues, accelerate circulation of blood and lymph fluid, and enhance the WBC and RBC counts in the blood consequently. This stimuli can also increase the oxygen demand of the peripheral tissues and increase the heart rate, the respiration frequency and oxygen intake rate of the lung in a unit time, so it has the effects of promoting flow of Qi and Blood and harmonizing the Defensive Qi and the Nutritive Qi.

(2) Relieving fatigue and enhancing the resistant ability of the body against diseases

Metabolic products will accumulate in the body when one is in activity. This will further cause a feeling of fatigue or discomfort due to reduce of energy reserved in muscles. If the emotion is in a depressive state in the case of fatigue, the feeling of discomfort will be aggravated.

By means of the regulatory effect of the channels, massage on foot can accelerate blood flow and the timely transportation of metabolic products, so it can bring about pleasure and ease to a person, increase one's adaptability, relieve fatigue and enhance the resistant ability of the human body against diseases.

(3) Treating inflammation, arresting pain and promoting tissue repairment

In terms of Western medicine, inflammatory pain is a manifestation of disturbance of circulation. In the case of inflammation, there exists difficult venous return, increased osmotic pressure and the resultant swelling in the local zone which will aggravate the disturbance of blood circulation, and substances which tend to irritate the tissues are likely to be produced. As massage on foot can accelerate the venous return in the local area, lower down the osmotic pressure and dissipate the inflammation, it has the effect of removing stagnancy and relieving pain. Massage on the points or reflecting zones in foot can also bring about a sedative effect, enhance the tolerance of the body to pain, relieve pain and promote flow of Qi and Blood, so it can eliminate the congealed blood, promote regeneration and repairment of tissues and enhance the therapeutic effects in the treatment of diseases.

(4) Promoting flow of Qi and Blood to regulate functional balance of organs

Reflecting zones and points exist in the soles. If the two feet are placed in a parallel position, the reflecting zones in the soles are just correspondent to the visceral organs in positions.

The three Yin channels of foot start at the feet and the three Yang channels of foot terminate in feet. These channels are closely related to the Zang-Fu organs and the segments of the channels on feet. Therefore, physiologic functions and pathologic changes of all the Zang-Fu organs of the human body can be transmitted to the feet through the channels. And thus, massage on foot can promote flow of Qi and Blood and regulate the functional balance of the body by sending relevant messages to the corresponding tissues and organs with certain manipulations.

When functional disturbance occurs in an organ, impulse produced by stimulating the reflecting zone of the organ on foot or nerve ending can be transmitted to the spinal neuron and further to the organ through the afferent nerves, so it can regulate the functions of the Zang-Fu organs.

(5) Regulating the whole body comprehenesively

Frequent physical exercise of the body can ensure the health of the body and increase the adaptability of the body. Although massage on foot is not the physical exercise itself, it can bring about the same effects as the exercise. As stimulation on certain reflecting zones and points on foot can directly regulate the related tissues and organs and increase the resistant ability of the body against disease, in fact it has the effect of regulating the whole body comprehensively.

2. Principles for massage on point-zone in feet

These principles are made based on the wholistic concept and the syndrome identification and corresponding treatment and are used to guide prevention and treatment of diseases and health preservation.

A pressing pain is felt when the reflecting zones or points on feet are pressed in the case of the functional activities of the Zang-Fu organs being normal. However, when diseases happen to the Zang-Fu organs, a prickly sensation will be produced in the reflecting zones or points of the feet. So, the most sensitive parts found in pressing the reflecting zones of feet should be taken as the stress in treating diseases. Each massage treatment should last 20~30 minutes and two treatments should be carried out a day.

The force exerted on manipulations varies with the different constitutions, illness conditions, sexes and the points or zones. In most cases, appropriate constant stimuli is of choice, but the stimulation may be strengthened in cases with acute pain with avoidance of injurying the foot. During the manipulation, doctor should observe the local and systemic response of the patients to ensure that the treatment is reliable and safe. To obtain satisfactory therapeutic effect, it is necessary to perform massage on the zones or points of foot constantly and master the combined use of these zones or points. Although this therapy has not any side or toxic effects, easy to carry out and suitable for different stages of many diseases, it is not a therapy suitable for all the diseases. Such cases as acute diseases, severe pain and haemorrhage, which are contraindicated for massage on foot, should be treated with other therapies according to their illness conditions lest the diseases be delayed.

Massage on the zones or points in foot should be carried out comprehensively on the left foot first, then the right foot, until the disease is cured.

3. Advantages of massage on point-zone of foot

(1) Wide indications

As the reflecting zones and points corresponding to all the Zang-Fu organs are distributed over the foot, massage on foot can be widely applied to treat diseases of the internal medicine, surgery, gynecology, pediatrics, dermatology and the eye, nose, throat and mouth, especially those marked by functional disturbance of nerves and the endocrine systems.

(2) Reliable and safe without any side or toxic effects

The purpose of massaging the zones or points on feet lies in improving the resistant ability of the human body against diseases and treating diseases actively. It has not any side or toxic effects on the human body and can prevent important organs from being impaired by the chemical drugs, so it is a safe and reliable therapy.

(3) Diagnosing disease early and treating diseases quickly

When discomfort in certain parts of the body just begins, the related reflecting zone will present an abnormal prickly feeling, suggesting that early diagnosis and treatment should be made. Often, the massage on foot can relieve a disease very quickly.

(4) Simple and easy to perform, spread and popularize

As massage on feet requires no medical instruments and is easy to learn and to apply, it may be carried out at any time and any place by patients themselves. Besides, this therapy may be stopped temporarily if patient has other things to do and resumed again after other things are completed. Furthermore, this therapy is suitable for patients of any ages or occupations, the distribution of the reflecting zones is easy to learn and remember, and the manipulations are simple and convenient to be applied, so, it can be widely spread and learned.

(5) Cultivating one's moral, enhancing therapeutic effects and preserving one's health

Anyone hopes that he or she has a full vigour, a healthy physique and a long life span. Massage on foot by oneself, which can keep fit, prevent and treat diseases, has the effect of prolonging life and thus is another way to health. As this therapy can be applied among the family members or freinds, and the family members have a good knowledge about the psychology, emotion and diseases of the patient, the patient and the family members can cooperate well in the treatment. As a matter of fact, love among the family members is a good drug for the patient's disease, and a patient can get rid of the psychological disorders with a pleasant and ease mind in the treatment. Therefore, massage on feet can cultivate one's moral, enhance the therapeutic effect and preserve ones health.

4. Commonly used manipulations in foot point-zone massage

Manipulations refer to the methods of exerting the treatments, which are various kinds. Clinically, they should be adopted in accordance with the illness conditions and the zones and points being treated. Several kinds of manipulations may be selected at the same time.

(1) Pushing

Manipulation: This is a method by exerting a stable force slowly and evenly through the belly of one finger or several fingers or the muscles of the thenar eminence or the hypothenar (Fig. 1). When this manipulation is applied, patient often has a feeling of hotness in the treating skin.

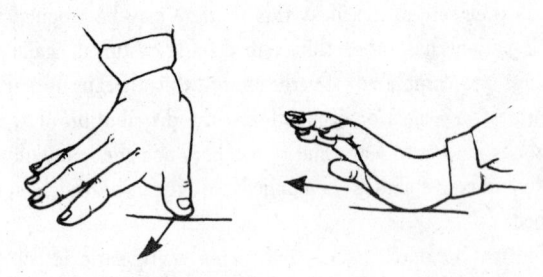

Fig. 1

Applications: The entire feet, mostly used when pressing the longitude lines or the toes towards different directions.

Indications: Relax muscles, activate Blood, relieve spasm, arrest pain, harmonize Defensive Qi and Nutritive Qi, and relieve fatigue.

(2) Kneading

Manipulation: This is a method marked by applying force softly, gently, slowly and semicircularly on a selected zone through the tip of the thumb, the index or the middle finger (Fig. 2). When it is applied, the finger exerting the force should move semicircularly together with the skin in the zone being treated so that an internal soft and slow friction can be arised between the skin and the tissues beneath. The hand doing the manipulation should adhere to the zone being treated and should avoid moving or rubbing on the surface of the skin. The frequency is between 100~160 times.

Applications: Suitable for the toes and the points in a broad area of the feet.

Indications: Regulate Qi and Blood, activate Blood flow and remove Blood Stasis, subdue swelling, relieve pain, warm up channels to dispel cold, and promote digestion.

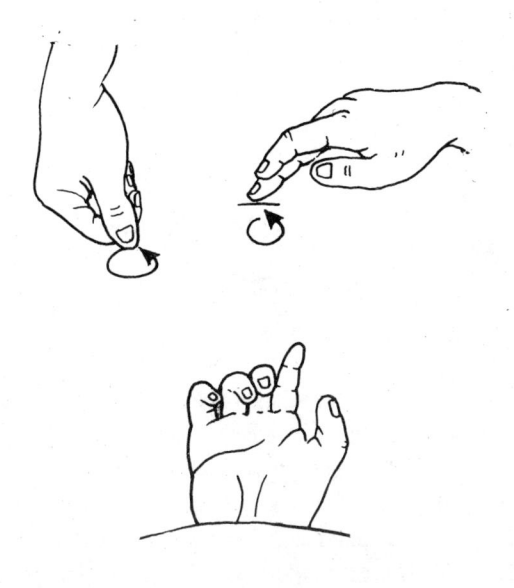

Fig. 2

(3) Pressing

Manipulation: This is a method marked by applying the force repeatedly on the points being treated through the tip of a finger or the palm in the order of exerting the force gentely first and then heavily and on the sallow part first and then the deeper part (Fig. 3). The force exerted should be stable and gradually strengthened. When the method reaches certain depth, the zone being pressed will present an obvious sorness and distending sensation, which indicates gaining of Qi. Then, the method is stopped at this depth for about 5~10 sec., and then the hand is raised slowly. This should be repeated about 10 times in each treatment, and clinically, pressing method is often adopted together with kneading manipulation, which is also known as pressing-kneading method.

Applications: All the zones and points on feet, mostly used on the points in a broad area of the feet.

Indications: Activate flow of Qi and Blood in the channels and collaterals, **regulate Yin and Yang,** promote digestion, remove Blood Stasis, subdue swelling and arrest pain.

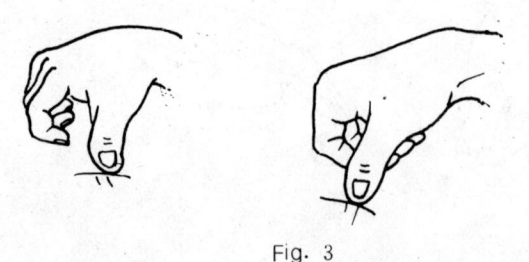

Fig. 3

(4) Pointing

Manipulation: This is a manipulation marked by applying powerful force on the deeper tissues of the human body through the tip of the thumb or the middle finger, or through the prominent part of the dorsal aspect of the proxysmal interphalangeal articulation of the flexed middle finger, the index finger and the thumb (Fig. 4). As this is a manipulation producing strong stimulation, the pressure exerted should be aggravated gradually so that patient has a strong feeling of gaining Qi. In clinical practice, it is usually used jointly with kneading manipulation, which is known as pointing-kneading manipulation.

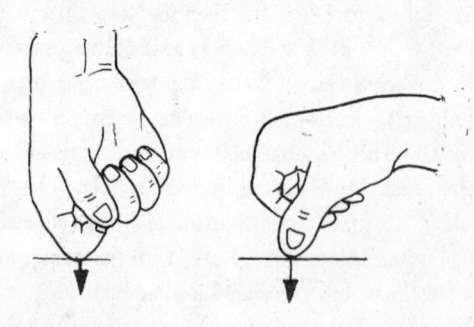

Fig. 4

Application: Mostly used in the small reflecting zone that requires strong stimulation or the points in the gaps of bones.

Indications: Promote flow of Qi and Blood in the channels and collaterals, activate Blood and remove Blood Stasis, subdue swelling and relieve pain.

(5) Rubbing

Manipulation: This is a manipulation marked by pushing and rubbing the selected area back and fro repeatedly along a line with a finger or with the thenar eminence or the hypothenar eminence touching the skin of the area closely (Fig. 5). The force exerted in this manipulation should be light but not floating and the back-fro movement should be quick until the patient feels warm or hot in the area being treated.

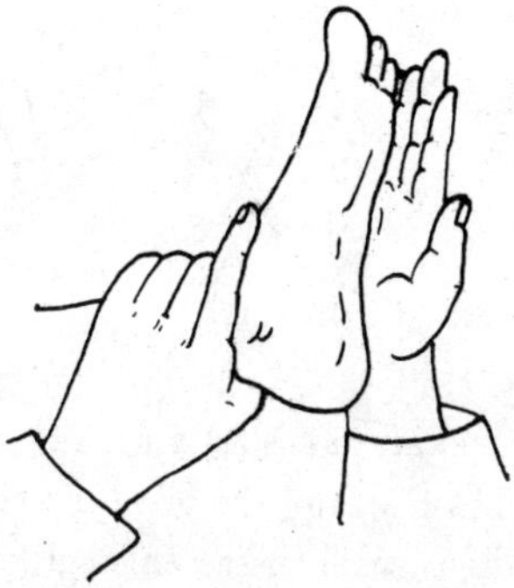

Fig. 5

Applications: Mostly used in the zones or points distributed along the longitude line of bones or in the soles or the centre of the soles.

Indications: Promote flow of Qi, activate Blood, warm and tonify the body, remove obstruction from the collaterals, dispel Cold, supplement Essence and marrow, prevent diseases, build up health and prevent ageing.

(6) Palm-rubbing

Manipulation: This is a manipulation marked by rubbing the skin of the reflecting zone clockwise or counterclockwise with the palm or the belly of the index finger, the middle finger or the ring finger touching the skin closely. This manipulation is softer and slower than the kneading manipulation, and it is required that the manipulation should be gentle and superficial at an even and coordinative speed so that the force exerted only reaches the skin and the subcutaneous area. The manipulation may start at the centre of the area and gradually to its surrounding area until patient has a feeling of warmth in the area being treated (Fig. 6).

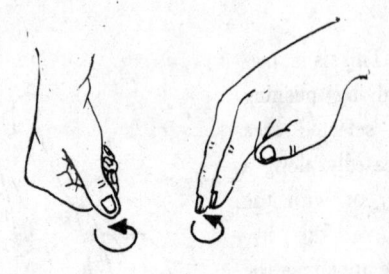

Fig. 6

Applications: Mostly applied in the points or reflecting zones in the broad area of the feet, especially suitable for diseases of young children, senile disease and chronic diseases. Usually the manipulation starts at the toes. It may also be used as a relaxing manipulation after a heavy manipulation is completed.

Indications: Warm up channels, dispel cold, promote flow of Qi and activate Blood, dissipate masses, relieve pain and remove obstruction from collaterals.

(7) Finger-nail pressing

This is a manipulation marked by pressing the points or reflecting zones through the distal border or the radial border of the nail of the thumb. It is a strong stimulating manipulation, so it should be done in a short time by exerting less strength first and then more strengthen and from the shallow to the deeper part. Be sure not to injury the skin (Fig. 7). In mostly cases, a

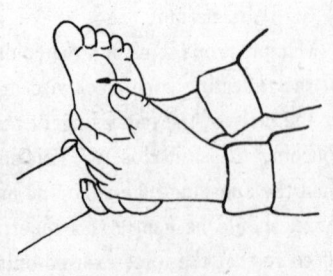

Fig. 7

strong sore and distending feeling is produced in the points or zones being pressed, and after the manipulation, the local zone should be mildly kneaded to alleviate the discomfort caused by the pressing.

Application: Mostly applied to the smaller zones such as the toes, junction of the toes and the gaps of the metatarcarpal bones. It is often adopted in combination with other manipulations simultaneously or alternatively.

Indications: Promote flow of Blood in the channels and collaterals, restore resuscitation and relieve mental depression.

(8) Rotating

Manipulation: Make the toes and the ankle joint do passive and gentle movement evenly and circularly (Fig. 8). When performing this manipulation, the operator should limit the movement within the normal physiological extent of the foot, the strength should be powerful and stable, changing from smaller to greater. The operator should perform the manipulation by fixing the patient's foot with one hand and rotating the foot with the other hand. Over strenous manipulation should be avoided lest the joint be injured.

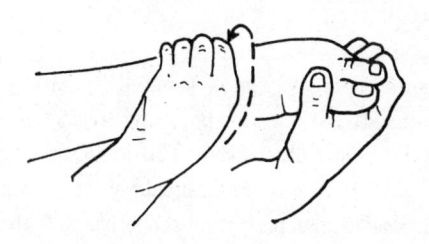

Fig. 8

Applications: Mostly applied in the toes or the ankle joints, used to treat chronic diseases, senile diseases, traumatic injury in a local zone and preserve one's health.

Indications: Relax the body, benefit the movement of the joints and keep the joint fexible.

(9) Holding and twisting

Manipulation: This is performed by holding a selected zone or point in the foot with the bellies of the thumb and the index finger and then twisting the zone or point lightly and evenly at a high speed. (Fig. 9). The manipulation should be light but not floating, heavy but not retaining.

Applications: Mainly applied to the toes, the small articulations of the foot, and the reflecting zones on the dorsum of feet, used to treat chronic diseases, discomfort in local zones and to keep health. It is also often used together with other manipulations such as finger-nail pressing and pushing.

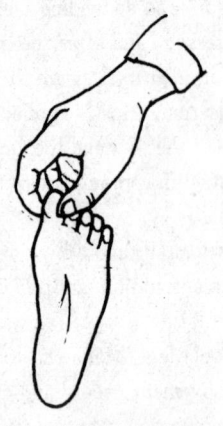

Fig. 9

Indications: Promote flow of Qi, activate circulation of Blood, benefit movement of joints, remove obstruction from the collaterals, relieve pain, dispel Wind, soften hard masses and dissipate nodules.

(10) Tracting

Manipulation: Fixing one end of a selected joint of the patient's foot with one hand, the operator pulls and tracts the other end of the joint with his or her other hand. This is known as tracting manipulation (Fig. 10). The operator should exert the strength along the longitude line of the foot joint properly, and the movement should be even, quick, flexible and harmonious. Application of strength at an angle with the line should be avoided lest the ligament and the joints be damaged.

Applications: Applied to the ankle joint, the interphalangeal joints, metatarsophalangeal joints, etc., used to treat senile diseases, local disorders of the joints of foot and to keep health. It may also be adopted in combination with other manipulations.

Indications: Activate Blood and remove obstruction from collaterals, benefit movement of joints, promote flow of Qi to relieve pain. It is a good way to relax the joints, and it can improve the movement extent of the joints.

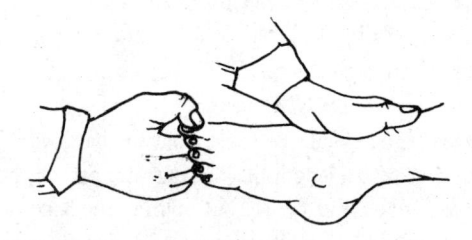

Fig. 10

5. The reducing and reinforcing effects of the manipulations

Application of different manipulations would produce different effects of reduction or reinforcement. Appropriate manipulations should be adopted according to the principles of "treating the Excess with reducing method, the Deficiency with reinforcing method, and a syndrome with both Deficiency and Excess with both the reducing method and the reinforcing method" (Table 1).

Table 1 Reducing and Reinforcing Manipulations

Classification Manipulation Techniques	Reinforce (the Deficiency Syndrome)	Reduce (the Excess Syndrome)
Massage along the distributive route of channel	Along the distributive direction	Against the distributive direction
Massage along the direction of blood flow	Centrically	Eccentrically
Manipulation directions	Clockwise	Counterclockwise
Manipulation strength	mild	great
Speed of the rhythm	low	great
Manipulation duration	Long	Short

6. Commonly used instruments and techniques in the foot point-zone massage

The above mentioned manipulations can be performed by a doctor or other persons, or by the patient himself. When some patients, especially the middle aged or the aged patients, have difficulty in bending their bodies to perform the foot massage themselves due to disturbance of movement or rigidity of the body, the following instruments and techniques should be adopted as a supplement according to their different conditions.

(1) Massage with massage rod

The massage rod should be made from the hard wood or plastics after being cut, with a length that the operator can touch his feet. It should be easily held tightly without injuring the hand or fall of the rod from the hand. Its thickiness should change gradually from great to small and its two ends should be rubbed into ball-shaped. The rod should be smooth and a soft rub pad should be used to cover the ball so that the skin is not damaged when the sole is massaged and the rod doesn't slide from the sole. This kind of rod can be used to massage most of the selected zones in the feet.

(2) Treading on glass balls with barefoot

Take a standing or sitting position. Tread several glass balls constantly with the balls touching the reflecting zones of the foot. When doing so, one should touch a fixed object with his hands to prevent himself from falling. 30 minutes each time, once or twice a day.

(3) Stepping a bamboo rod

Place a bamboo rod flat on the ground, then step the rod with a barefoot with the rod touching the pathologic reflecting zones. 30 minutes each time, once or twice daily.

(4) Stepping the crossbeam of a stool

In a sitting position, step on the crossbeam of a stool or chair or a magnetic massagor to stimulate the pathological reflecting zones or points of feet. 30 minutes each time, once or twice daily.

7. Attentions for foot point-zone massage

The massage room should be kept clean and tide, free from wind, strong light or stimuli of noise. The air in the room should be fresh, and the general environment should be kept comfortable.

The operator must have a lofty medical ethics, a strong physique, a good tolerance and a good knowledge of the selected zones or points.

Tell the patient to wash his feet with warm water before the treatment, relax his body and his mind completely, and lie flat a while in bed. Then, the operator takes a sitting position and place a bowl on his knees. After that, put the patient's feet over his knees and tell the patient the attentions so that the patient can cooperate well with the operator in the treatment.

The operator's hands and nails should be clean. Those with skin disorders are not allowed to perform the treatment in order to prevent contamination of the skin diseases and bring danger to patient.

Before pressing each of the pathologic zones or points, the operator should, firstly, find the points which produce a prickling pain on pressing so that the treatment is more specific and a better therapeutic effect can be obtained.

The strength exerted on massage should vary with the patient's constitutions, their illness conditions, and the requirements of the manipulations suitable for the selected zones or points.

It is advised to do the treatment at a regular time everyday, and the treatment should last $20 \sim 30$ minutes each time, once or twice daily.

After each treatment, patient should feel thirst and drink a cup of warm water within 30 minutes after the treatment. The aged and the young patients should drink less according to their different conditions.

If the patient presents any unfavorable reaction, the treatment should be stopped at once to ensure that the treatment is safe and reliable.

If patient presents fever, aversion to cold or tiredness after the treatment which are patient's normal response, he or she should continue the treatment.

After finishing one treatment, the operator should wash his or her hands with warm water and record the process of the treatment in order to observe the therapeutic effect and summarize experience.

8. Restraint for foot point-zone massage

Such conditions as skin ulcer, bleeding or infectious skin diseases occurring on the points or zones of feet should be treated first. Massage is prohibited strictly during the onset stage of the diseases.

Massage is prohibited strictly in patients with various kinds of tuberculosis of the joints, medullitis, bone tumor or fracture.

Generally, foot massage is prohibited in patients with severe cardiopathy, hypertension, schizophrenia and liver or kidney diseases unless as a first aid.

Foot massage cannot be adopted in cases with various kinds of acute or chronic infectious diseases, the haemorrhagic period of peptic ulcer or gastric preforation to prevent the diseases from being delayed.

Manipulation are not suggested during the pregnancy or menstruation to prevent abortion or excessive bleeding. The zones or points related to treatment of gynecological diseases, in particular, must be free from being pressed violently.

Massage on zones or points of feet are strictly prohibited in patients with hemopathy or a tendency to bleed, in order to prevent bleeding of the local zones.

Massage on the zones or points in feet is also prohibited in patients with an empty stomach. Usually the massage can be resumed 1 or 2 hours later after meal in these patients.

Structure and Function of Foot, Important Points and Reflecting Zones

*F*oot massage therapy is applied to the different parts of the foot and its adjacent tissues based on the meridian theory and the reflecting zones of the different parts of the human body. So, it is very important to have a good knowledge of the basic structure and function of the foot, master the location, manipulation and indication of the foot reflecting zones and the commonly adopted points of meridians located in the lower parts of the human body.

1. Structure and function of foot

A foot of a normal person consists of 26 bones, which are connected with each other by the ligaments, muscles and fibers (Fig. 11). Numerous branches of nerves, nerve ends and receptors exist in foot with abundant blood circulation (Fig. 12).

To meet the needs of the functions, there is a thick layer of fat and an arc, which is a structure unique to human body, in the feet. The arc of foot is a variable structure which changes with the position and posture of the body. It serves as a plastic "instrument" for the standing, walking and bearing of heavy things of the human body. It is an upright arc composed by the tarsal bone and the metatarsal bone by means of ligaments and joints. The arc of foot includes the longitude arc and the transverse arc and it can slow down and reduce the shock of the ground on the internal organs and tissues of the human body to protect these organs and tissues from being injuried. Meanwhile, it can also prevent the vessels and nerves on the soles from being pressed, thus it is a necessary structure for the human body to stand long, bear load or walk. Therefore, protection of the foot arc is very important to the human body.

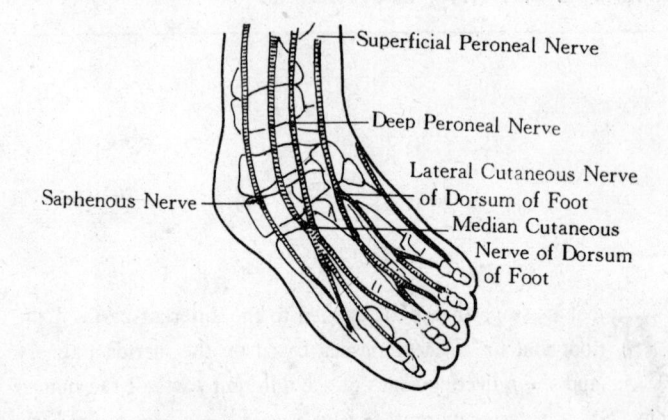

Fig. 11

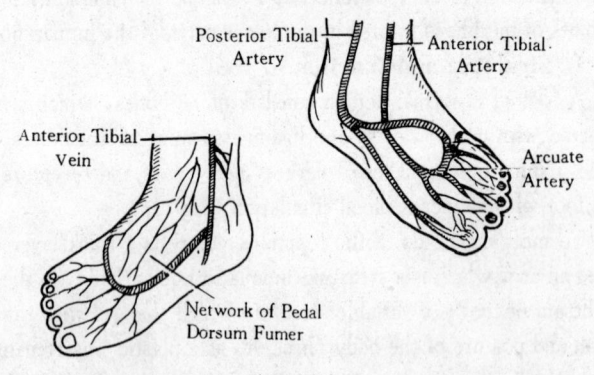

Fig. 12

Although the feet are in the lowest position of the human body, they are closely related to the head, hands and the organs and tissues in the body cavities. The numerous nerve ends in the feet communicate with the brain closely and the main channels originate from the feet. Response of feet to environmental temperature may cause corresponding reactions of the circulatory system, the digestive system and the respiratory system, and ageing and diseases of the human body often start at the feet. Clinical practice has proved that foot exercise could build up the constitution, treat diseases, postpone ageing and keep one in health.

2. Channels of foot

A number of points of the six foot channels of the twelve regular channels are located at feet according to the channel theory.

(1) The Stomach Channel of Foot-Yangming

This channel terminates at the lateral side of the second toe of the feet and is indicated for diseases of the digestive tract, the head, the face, the eyes, the nose, the mouth, the ears and the throat, such as gastric diseases, enteritis, dysentery, indigestion, appendicitis, headache, facial paralysis, eye diseases, toothache, mumps, inflammation of the pharynx and larynx and mastitis.

(2) The Gallbladder Channel of Foot-Shaoyang

This channel passes the external malleolus inferoanteriorly and terminates at the tip of the fourth toe. Its branch reaches the lateral side of the big toe after branching off at the dorsum of foot. It is indicated for diseases of the head and the lateral sides of the body, such as headache, deafness, tinnitus, eye diseases, hepatitis, cholecystitis, and diseases of the hypochondrium and the lateral sides of the legs.

(3) The Bladder Channel of Foot-Taiyang

This channel passes through the lateral side of the dorsum of foot and ends at the tip of the small toe, indicated for eye diseases, diseases of the head, nape, back, loins, sacrum and the posterior aspect of the legs, schizophrenia, epilepsy, and the diseases of the tissues and organs related to distribution of the channel.

(4) The Spleen Channel of Foot-Taiyin

This channel starts at the medial end of the great toe, mainly indicated for diseases of the digestive tract and the urinary and reproductive systems, such as stomachache, indigestion, dysentery, diarrhea, irregular menstruation, dysmenorrhea, retention of urine, and enuresis.

(5) The Liver Channel of Foot-Jueyin

This channel starts at the upper surface of the great toe, mainly indicated for diseases of the external genitalia, lower abdomen, liver and gallbladder and diseases of the head, such as headache, dizziness, facial paralysis, eye diseases, epilepsy, infection of the biliary tract, hepatitis, pain in the hypochondrium, dysmenorrhea, infection of the urinary system, and testitits.

(6) The Kidney Channel of Foot-Shaoyin

This channel starts below the little toe, then goes obliquely, passing the centre of sole and the inferior border of the pisi formis. It is mainly indicated for diseases of the urinary system and the reproductive system. It is also indicated for diseases of the respiratory system. Diseases that can be treated by selecting the points of the channel include emission, impotence, premature ejaculation, edema, retention of urine, enuresis, chronic lumbago, sore throat, toothache, insomnia, dizziness, tinnitus, decline of vision, etc.

The twelve regular channels interiorly pertain to Zang-Fu organs which have an interior-exterior relationship, so the Yin channels and the Yang channels are also interior-exteriorly related. That is, the Stomach Channel of Foot-Yangming is interior-exteriorly related to the Spleen Channel of Foot-Taiyin; the Bladder Channel of Foot-Taiyang is interior-exteriorly related to the Kidney Channel of Foot-Shaoyin; and the Gallbladder Channel is interior-exteriorly related to the Liver Channel of Foot-Jueyin. The two channels interior-exteriorly related are closely related to each other in physiology, influence each other in pathology and supplement to each other in treatment.

The trends of distribution of the six channels reaching the feet are that the three Yang channels of the foot go from the head to the feet and the three Yin channels of the foot run from the feet to the chest and abdomen. Apart from the points on the regular channels, many extra points exist in the feet. The twelve regular channels, distributed criss-crossely, travelling to both the interior and the exterior of the body and both the upper part and the lower part of the body, connect with the Zang-Fu organs. The eight extraordinary channels run across the twelve regular channels. So, all the Zang-Fu organs and tissues of the human body are coordinatively connected. The channels and the collaterals function to carry Qi and Blood, nourish the whole body, defend against pathogens and protect the human body. Each of the channels is distributed over a certain route and pertains to an organ and connect with another organ, so it can treat diseases of a local zone the channel passes through, the adjacent tissues on the route of the channels and the related internal Zang-Fu organs. Besides, one point of channels may influence the functions of a number of Zang-Fu organs, and one physiological function can be influenced by many points. Furthermore, the points of channels have a two-way regulatory effect on the human body. In other words, stimulation on the same point in different physiological states may bring about completely opposite therapeutic effects. When the function of the human body is hyperactive, the stimulation can inhibit the hyperactivity; while if the function is hypoactive, the stimulation can excite the hypoactivity. This kind of regulatory effect has influence not only on the local zones of the human body, but also on all the functional systems of the human body such as the defending function and the immunological function of the human body. Clinically, diseases can be generalized as those of a certain channel according to their different manifestations and distribution of the channels and the Zang-Fu organs the channels connect with. The related points or zones in feet can be used separately or in combination. See Table 2 and Table 3 for indications of the six channels of feet.

Table 2 Difference and Common Points of
the Three Yin Channels of Foot

	Feature	Common Points
The Foot Jueyin Channel	Diseases of the reproductive system, liver disease, gallbladder diseases and diseases of head or face	Diseases of the urinary and reproductive systems
The Foot Taiyin Channel	Diseases of the digestive system	
The Foot Shaoyin Channel	Diseases of the urinary, repoductive or respiratory systems	

Table 3 Difference and Common Points of
the Three Yang Channels of Foot

	Feature	Common Points
The Foot Yangming Channel	Diseases of the forehead, face, larynx, breasts and the gastrointestinal tract	Eye disease and febrile diseases
The Foot Shaoyang Channel	Diseases of the bilateral sides of head, ear, hypochondrium, liver and gallbladder	
The Foot Taiyang Channel	Diseases of the head, nape, back, lumbar region and sacral region (Points in the back treat diseases of their corresponding organs)	

The main points selected in the massage of foot point-zone include the five Shu points, the Yuan-Primary points, the Luo-Connecting points, the Xi-Cleft point, the crossing points, the eight Confluential points, the extra points and the experiential points. This is because that these points occupy a very important position in treatment of diseases, having very good effectiveness for the functions of the Zang-Fu organs, tendons, bones, Blood and vessels as well as many diseases. For example, the Jing-Well points are extremely effective for epigastric fullness; the Ying-Spring points for fever, the Shu-Stream points for arthralgia with heaviness of the body; the Jing-River points for cough, asthma, fever and chills; and the He-Sea points for adverse flow of Qi with diarrhea and diseases of the Fu organs. The Yuan-Primary points are usually adopted to treat diseases of the Zang organs; the Luo-Connecting points are most commonly used to treat diseases of the channel and the Zang-Fu organs related to the channels these points pertain to, and the Xi-Cleft channels are chiefly employed in the treatment of acute diseases of the Zang or Fu organs related to the channels the points pertain to. For example, Liangqiu, the Xi-Cleft point of the Stomach channel, can relieve acute stomach pain markedly. The eight confluential points have special effectiveness on some specific functional systems. For example, Yanglingquan, the confluential points of tendons, is a point that is always used in treatment of diseases of the tendons and muscles of the body. The crossing points are the points where several channels converge, so they can be used to treat diseases of the channels meeting at the points and the diseases of the Zang-Fu organs related to these channels. Sanyinjiao, for example, is where three Yin channels meet, so it can be adopted to treat diseases of the Liver, the Spleen and the Kidney channels. In addition, some points of channels are also specially effective for some diseases although they are not the above mentioned specific points. For instance, Xuehai, which is where Blood converges, has the effects of strengthening the Spleen, inducing diuresis and harmonizing Ying-Blood, so it can be used to treat various kinds of gynecological diseases and skin diseases. The extra points and the experiential points are the points with special effects not located on the fourteen channels. For example, Duyin point can treat intolerable cardiac pain.

3. Important points in foot

(1) Important points of the Stomach Channel of Foot-Yangming (Fig. 13)

① Liangqiu (Xi-Cleft point)

Locations: 2 cun above the superiolateral border of the petalla.

Indications: Gastric pain, mastitis, numbness, muscular atrophy and pain of the knee joint and the anterior aspect of the lower leg.

② Zusanli (He-Sea point)

Location: 3 cun below the external Xiyan, one finger breadth lateral to the anterior crest of the tibia.

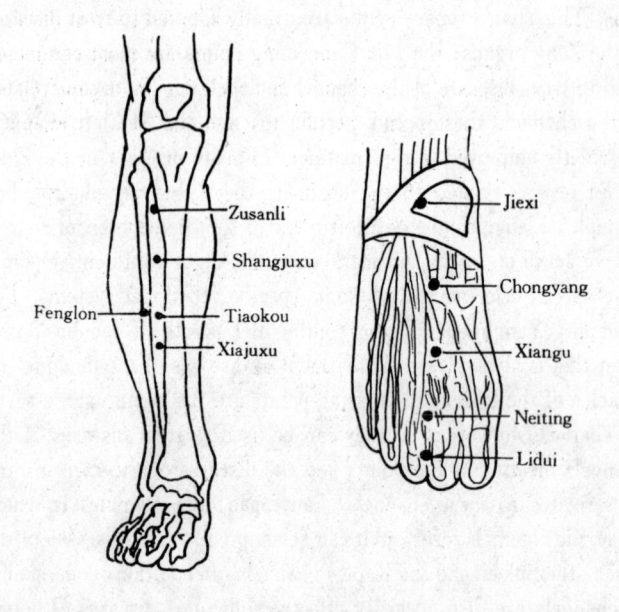

Fig. 13

Indications: Mainly the diseases of the gastrointestinal tract, such as gastric pain, vomiting, diarrhea, dysentery and appendicitis, diseases of the liver and gallbladder, insomnia, hypertension, shock, fever, indigestion, beriberi, edema, numbness and flaccidity of the lower limbs. It also has the effect of preserving health and improving constitution.

③ Shangjuxu (Lower He-Sea point)

Location: 3 cun directly below Zusanli.

Indication: Appendicitis, acute or chronic diarrhea, and numbness and flaccidity of the lower limbs.

④ Tiaokou

Location: 2 cun below Shangjuxu.

Indication: Shoulder periarthritis and systremma.

⑤ Fenglong (Luo-Connecting point)

Location: One finger breadth lateral to Tiaokou.

Indications: Cough with profuse sputum, asthma, dizziness, schizophrenia, epilepsy, and numberness, pain and muscular atrophy of the lateral side of the lower limbs.

⑥ Jiexi (Jing-River point)

Location: On the dorsum of foot, at the midpoint of the transverse crease of the ankle, between the tendon of long extensor muscle of great toe and the tendon of the long extensor muscle of the toe.

Indications: Headache, nephritis, enteritis, epilepsy, indigestion, abdominal fullness, constipation, diseases of the peripheral soft tissues of the ankle and drop foot.

⑦ Chongyang (Yuan-Source point)

Location: Below Jiexi, in the highest point of the dorsum of foot, between the 2nd metarcarpal bone and the cuneiform bone where the pedal doral artery is felt.

Indications: Headache, facial paralysis, toothache, pain in dorsum of foot, malaria, schizophrenia, and febrile diseases.

⑧ Xiagu (Shu-Stream point)

Location: On the dorsum of foot, in the depression anterior to the junction of the 2nd and 3rd metarcarpal bones.

Indications: Edema of face, conjunctivitis, edema, borborygmus and abdominal pain, and hysteria.

⑨ Neiting (Ying-Spring point)

Location: On the dorsum of foot, between the 2nd and the 3rd toes, at the junction of the white and red skin posterior to the border of web.

Indications: Toothache, trigerminal neuralgia, tonsilitis, gastric pain, acid regurgitation, abdominal distension, diarrhea, acute or chronic enteritis, dysentery, hernia, beriberi, etc.

⑩ Lidui (Jing-Well point)

Location: In the lateral side of the proximal metacarpal bone of the 2nd toe, 0.1 cun away from the corner of nail.

Indications: Brain ischemia, neurosism, tonsilitis, facial paralysis, hepatitis, indigestion, epistaxis and hysteria.

(2) Important points of the Bladder Channel of Foot-Taiyang

(Fig. 14)

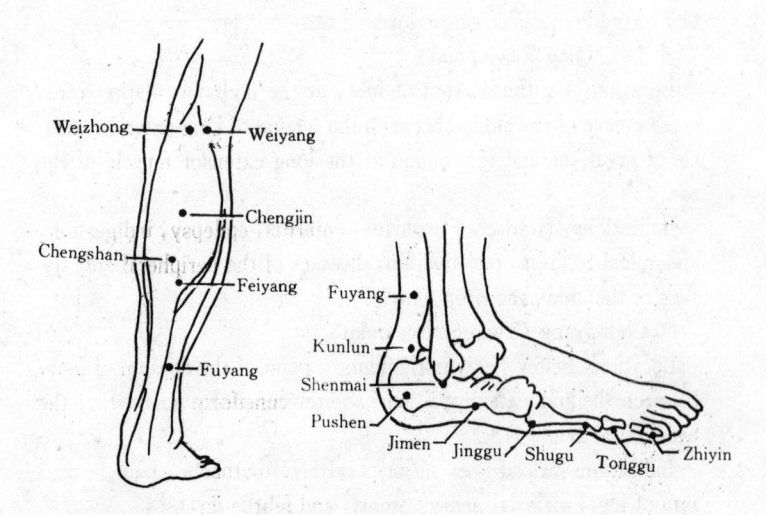

Fig. 14

① Weiyang (Lower He-Sea point of Triple-Jiao)

Location: In the lateral end of the transverse crease of the popliteal fossa and the medial border of the tendon of biceps muscle of thigh.

Indications: Nephritis, cystitis, chyluria, abdominal distension, dysuria, enuresis, hemorrhoid, rigidity and pain in the back and lumbar region, convulsion of leg and foot, paralysis of the lower limbs, etc.

② Weizhong (He-Sea point)

Location: In the midpoint of the transverse crease of popliteal fossa.

Indications: Acute rigidity and pain in the back and lumbar region, sciatica, systremma, numbness, pain or paralysis in the lower limbs, epilepsy, heat-stroke, epistaxis, boil, eczema, anal itching, mastitis, sore throat, vomiting, diarrhea, acute gastroenteritis, etc.

③ Chengshan

Location: Between the two bellies of the gastrocnemius muscles, in the depression of the tip of the " ∧ " shaped crease of the posterior aspect of the lower leg when the tips of toes are extended straight with force.

Indications: Sciatica, systremma, pain in the sacral and lumbar region, atrophy of the gastreocnemius muscles, paralysis of the lower limbs, constipation, diarrhea, prolapse of rectum, hemorrhoid, beriberi, infantile convulsion or epilepsy, and heel pain.

④ Feiyang (Luo-Connecting Point)

Location: 7 cun directly above Kunlun, in the lateroinferior aspect of Chengshan.

Indications: Soreness of loins and knees, heaviness and pain of the lower limbs, sciatica, hemorrhoid, headache and pain in the nape, vertigo, nasal obstruction, epistaxis, nephritis, cystitis, etc.

⑤ Fuyang (Xi-Cleft point)

Location: 3 cun directly above Kunlun.

Indications: Headache, heaviness of the head, rigidity and pain in the nape, back, sacral region and lumbar region, fever and chills with convulsion, beriberi, paralysis and numbness of lower limbs, sciatica, etc.

⑥ Kunlun (Jing-Stream point)

Location: In the posterior aspect of the external malleolus, in the depression between the tip of the external malleolus and the heel.

Indications: Headache, rigidity of neck, goiter, pain in the back and lower back, sciatica, paralysis of lower limbs, diseases of the ankles and their sorrounding soft tissues, epistaxis, distocia, retained labor, etc.

⑦ Pushen

Location: In the laterior side of the foot, posteroinferior to the external malleolus, directly below Kunlun, lateral to heel, and at the junction of the white and red skin.

Indications: Lumbago, heel pain, paralysis of lower limbs, beriberi, epilepsy and schizophrenia.

⑧ Shenmai (One of the eight confluential points, communicating with Yangqiao channel)

Location: In the lateral side of the foot, in the depression directly below the external malleolus.

Indications: Headache, cerebrospinal meningitis, auditory vertigo, epilepsy, schizophrenia, arthritis of the ankle, pain in the loins and knees.

⑨ Jinmen (Xi-Cleft point)

Location: In the lateral side of the foot, directly below the anterior border of the external malleolus.

Indications: Epilepsy, infantile convulsion, pain in the lumbar region and legs, pain in the sole, toothache, headache and deafness.

⑩ Jinggu (Yuan-Primary point)

Location: In the lateral side of foot, posteroinferior to the 5th metatarsal bone, at the junction of the white and red skin.

Indications: Myocarditis, meningitis, epilepsy, pain in the lumbar region and legs, headache and rigidity of nape.

⑪ Shugu (Shu-Stream point)

Location: In the lateral side of foot, posterior to the 5th metatarsophalangeal joint, at the junction of white and red skin.

Indications: Pain in the head and nape, malaria, eye nebula, epilepsy, schizophrenia, dysentery and hemorrhoid.

⑫ Zutonggu (Ying-Spring point)

Location: In the lateral side of foot, anterior to the 5th metatarsophalangeal joint, at the junction of the white and red skin.

Indications: Headache, vertigo, asthma, epistaxis, schizophrenia, and congestion of uterus.

⑬ Zhiyin (Jing-Well Point)

Location: In the lateral side of the distal segment of the little toe, 0.1 cun away from the corner of nail.

Indications: Headache, pain of eye, nasal obstruction, epistaxis, apoplexy, improper fetal position, distocia, emission, etc.

(3) Important points of the Gallbladder Channel of Foot-Shaoyang (Fig. 15)

① Yanglinquan (He-Sea point and the confluential point of the tendon)

Location: In the depression inferoanterior to the head of fibula.

Indications: Diseases of the liver and gallbladder such as hepatitis, cholecystitis, ascariasis of the biliary tract and jaundice, vomiting, bitter taste in the mouth and pain in the hypochondric region, hemiplegia, paralysis of the lower limbs, sciatica, paralysis of the fibular nerve, trauma of the knee joint and its adjacent soft tissues, etc.

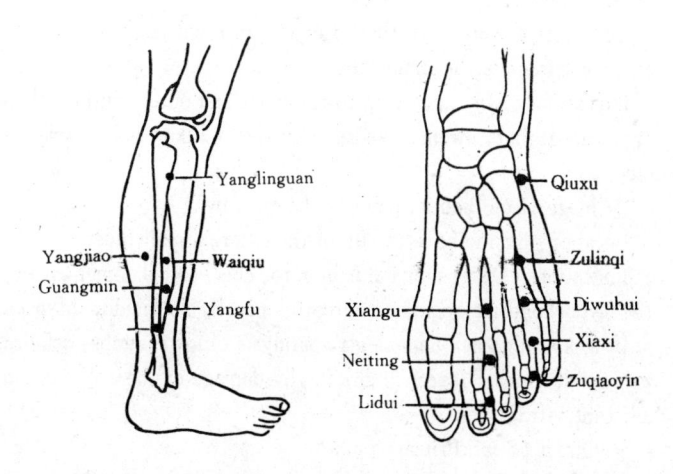

Fig. 15

② Yangjiao (Xi-Cleft point)

Location: 7 cun above the tip of the external malleolus, on the posterior border of the fibula.

Indications: Cholecystitis, intercostal neuralgia, fullness and distension in the chest and hypochondrium, mania, epilepsy, schizophrenia, aphasia, sore throat, beriberi, pain in the knee, paralysis of the lower limbs, systremma, sciatica, etc.

③ Waiqiu (Xi-Cleft point)

Location: 7 cun above the tip of the external malleolus, on the anterior border of the fibula.

Indications: Headache, stiff neck, sciatica, paralysis of lower limbs, hepatitis, cholecystitis, fullness in the hypochondriac region, epilepsy with foamy spittle, beriberi, etc.

④ Guangming (Luo-Connecting point)

Location: 5 cun above the tip of the external malleolus, on the anterior border of the fibula.

Indications: Myopia, night blindness, optic atrophy, decline of eye vision in the aged, migraine, schizophrenia, epilepsy, mastitis, distending pain of breast and paralysis of the lower limbs.

⑤ Yangfu (Jing-Well point)

Location: 4 cun above the tip of the external malleolus, on the anterior border of the fibula.

Indications: Migraine, pain in the inner and outer canthus of the eye, sore throat, swelling and pain in the auxillary fossa, sciatica, etc.

⑥ Juegu (Confluential point of the marrow)

Location: 3 cun above the tip of the external malleolus.

Indications: Distension and pain in the chest and abdomen, pain in the hypochondriac region, intercostal neuralgia, rigidity of neck, stiff neck, migraine, hemiplegia, paralysis of lower limbs, sciatica, pain in the lateral aspect of the thigh, damage of the ankle and its adjacent soft tissues.

⑦ Qiuxu (Yuan-Primary point)

Location: Inferoanterior to the external malleolus, in the depression lateral to the tendon of the long extensor muscle of toes.

Indications: Pain in the hypochondriac region, cholecystitis, tuberculosis of the lymph node in the auxillary fossa, sciatica, diseases of the ankle and its surrounding soft tissues, paralysis of the lower limbs and hernia.

⑧ Zulinqi (Shu-Stream point)

Location: In the lateral aspect of the dorsum, in the depression anterior to the junction of the 4th and the 5th metatarsal bones.

Indications: Headache, dizziness, conjunctivitis, mastitis, tuberculosis of the cervical lymph nodes, pain in the hypochondriac region, foot pain, suppression of lactation, irregular menstruation and diseases of the biliary tract.

⑨ Xiaxi (Ying-Spring point)

Location: In the lateral side of the dorsum, between the 4th and the 5th toes, at the junction of the white and red skin posterior to the web.

Indications: Migraine, hypertension, tinnitus, deafness, intercostal neuralgia, mastitis, edema of limbs, general migratory pain, paralysis of lower limbs and hot sensation in the soles.

⑩ Zuqiaoyin (Jing-Well point)

Location: In the lateral side of the distal segment of the 4th toe, 0.1 cun distal to the corner of nail.

Indications: Headache, hypertension, conjunctivitis, intercostal neuralgia, asthma, pleuritis, hiccup, neurosis, irregular menstruation and coma.

(4) Important points of the Kidney Channel of Foot-Shaoyin (Fig. 16)

① Yongquan (Jing-Well point)

Location: In the sole, in the depression of the anterior part of the foot when the foot is bent, at the junction of the anterior 1/3 and the posterior 2/3 of the sole.

Indications: Shock, sun-stroke, insomnia, apoplexy, headache, dizziness, hypertension, epilepsy, hysteria, schizophrenia, infantile convulsion, pain in the vertex, paralysis of lower limbs, dry mouth with less fluid, diabetes, asthma, hematemesis, palpitation, irregular menstruation, deafness, tinnitus, prolapse of uterus, sterility, emission, impotence and dry and cracked foot.

② Rangu (Ying-Spring point)

Location: In the medial border of foot, at the junction of the white and red skin inferior to the tubersity of the navicular bone.

Indications: Pharygnitis, laryngitis, cystitis, irregular menstruation, diabetes, tetanus, newborn tetanus, diarrhea, leukorrhagia, emission and diseases of the heart and lung.

③ Taixi (Shu-Stream and Yuan-Primary point)

Location: In the medial side of the foot, posterior to the medial malleolus, in the depression between the tip of the medial malleolus and the heel.

Indications: Nephritis, cystitis, irregular menstruation, emission, enuresis, toothache, chronic laryngitis, tinnitus, emphysema, neurosis, lumbago, paralysis of lower limbs, pain in the soles, constipation, and fall of hair.

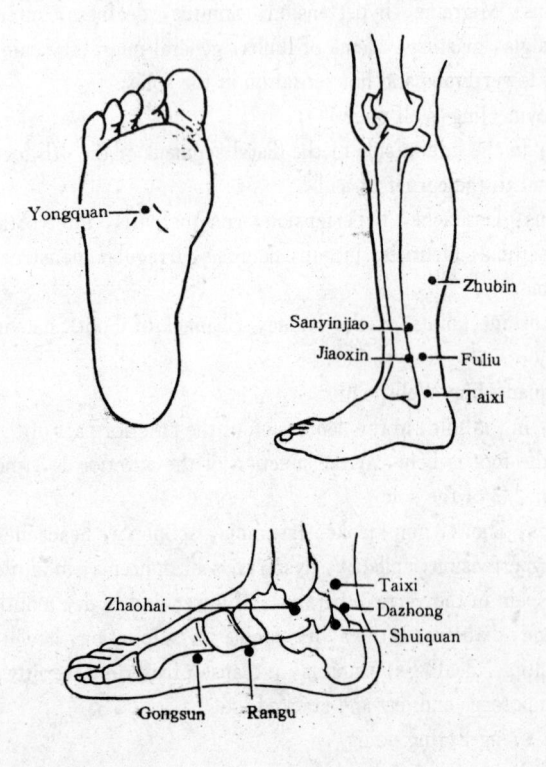

Fig. 16

④ Dazhong (Luo-Connecting point)

Location: In the medial side of foot, posteroinferior to medial malleolus, in the depression anterior to the attachment of the heel.

Indications: Asthma, malaria, neurosis, hysteria, retention of urine, sore throat, heel pain, dementia, toothache, and neuralgia in the lumbar region.

⑤ Shuiquan (Xi-Cleft point)

Location: In the medial side of foot, 1 cun directly below Taixi, in the depression medial to the tuberosity of the calcaneus.

Indications: Amenorrhea, prolapse of uterus, myopia, irregular menstruation and dysmenorrhea.

⑥ Zhaohai (One of the eight confluential points, communicating with Yinqiao Channel)

Location: In the medial side of foot, in the depression inferior to the tip of the medial malleolus.

Indications: Pharyngitis, laryngitis, tonsilitis, neurosis, hysteria, epilepsy, irregular menstruation, prolapse of uterus, leukorrhagia and constipation.

⑦ Fuliu (Jing-Stream point)

Location: 2 cun above Taixi, in the anterior border of the calcaneus.

Indications: Spontaneous sweating, night sweating, emission, impotence, edema, abdominal fullness, borborygmus, diarrhea, dry throat, hemorrhoid, nephritis, infection of urinary tract, dysfunctional uterine bleeding, paralysis of lower limbs, etc.

⑧ Zhubin (Xi-Cleft point of Yinwei Channel)

Location: 5 cun directly above Taixi.

Indications: Pain in the lower abdomen, hernia, epilepsy, mania, schizophrenia, menorrhage, pelvic inflammation, nephritis, cystitis, infection of urinary tract and pain in the lower leg.

⑨ Yingu (He-Sea point)

Location: In the medial side of the transverse crease of the popliteal fossa and between the semi-tendinous and semi-membranous muscles when the knee is flexed.

Indications: Impotence, emission, hernia, metrostaxis and metrorrhagia, menorrhagia, infection of the urinary tract, retention of urine, mania, dampness and itching in the scrotum, and pain in the medial side of the thigh and knee joint.

(5) Important Points of the Liver Channel of Foot-Jueyin (Fig. 17)

① Dadun (Jing-Well Point)

Location: 0.1 cun lateral to the corner of the nail of great toe.

Indications: Testitis, prolapse of uterus, irregular menstruation, hernia with pain, hematuria, metrostaxis and metrorrhagia, epilepsy, eczema of scrotum, swelling, pain and redness of eyes, etc.

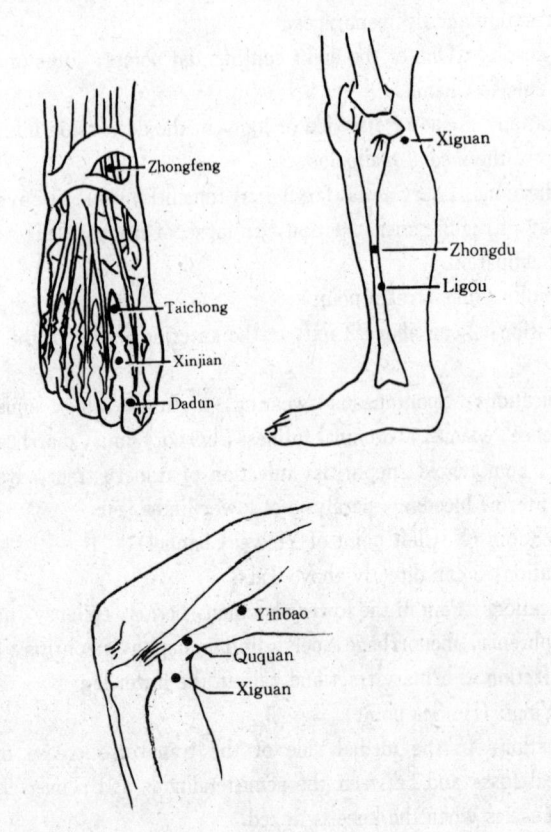

Fig. 17

② Xingjian (Ying-Spring point)

Location: On the dorsum of foot, between the 2nd and 3rd toes, at the junction of the white and red skin posterior to the web.

Indications: Headache, dizziness, glaucoma, intercostal neuralgia, testitis, hernia, menorrhagia, infantile convulsion, night sweat, epilepsy, dysmenorrhea, leukorrhagia, apoplexy and pain of the knee joint.

③ Taichong (Yuan-Primary and Yuan-Source point)

Location: On the dorsum of foot, in the depression anterior to the junction of the 1st and 2nd metatarsal bones.

Indications: Headache, dizziness, hypertension, insomnia, hepatitis, mastitis, irregular menstruation, thrombopenia, aching of limb joints and infantile convulsion.

④ Zhongfeng (Jing-Well point)

Location: On the dorsum of foot, anterior to the medial malleolus, at the midpoint of the line connecting Shangqiu and Jiexi, in the depression of the anterior tendon of the tibia.

Indications: Hepatitis, retention of urine, emission, pain of penis, hernia, lower abdominal pain, and diseases of the ankle and its adjacent soft tissues.

⑤ Ligou (Luo-Connecting point)

Location: 5 cun above the medial malleolus, in the center of the medial aspect of the tibia.

Indications: Irregular menstruation, metrostaxis and metrorrhagia, leukorrhagia, swelling and pain of testis, dysuria, enuresis, hernia, inflammation of pelvic cavity and abdominal fullness.

⑥ Zhongdu (Xi-Cleft point)

Location: 2 cun directly above Ligou.

Indications: Abdominal pain, diarrhea, metrostaxis and metrorrhagia, hernia, paralysis of lower limbs, etc.

⑦ Ququan (He-Sea point)

Location: In the depression of the medial end of the transverse crease of the knee joint when the knee is flexed.

Indications: Prolapse of uterus, pain in the lower abdomen, dysuria, enuresis, pain and itching of the external genitalia, emission, impotence, diarrhea, nephritis, hypertension, prostatitis, and swelling and pain in the medial aspect of the knee joint.

(6) Important Points of the Spleen Channel of Foot-Taiyin (Fig. 18)

① Yinbai (Jing-Well point)

Location: In the medial side of the distal segment of the great toe, 0.1 cun away from the corner of nail.

Indications: Menorrhagia, bleeding of digestive tract, abdominal pain, abdominal fullness, schizophrenia, hemafecia, hematuria, acute enteritis and dream-disturbed sleep.

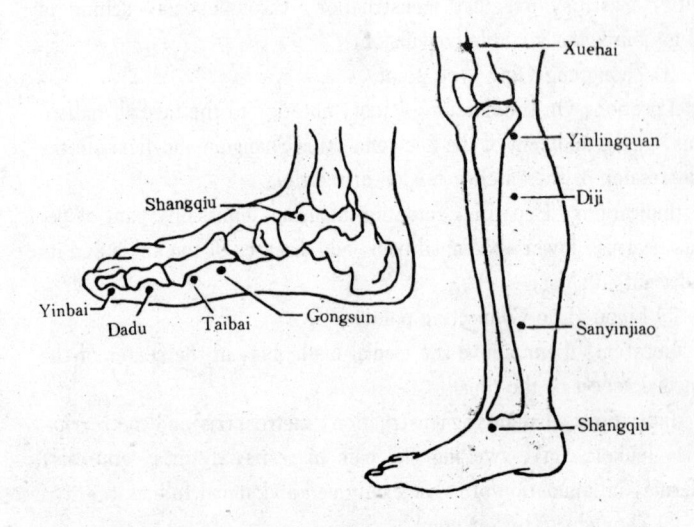

Fig. 18

② Dadu (Ying-Spring point)

Location: In the medial side of the foot, in the depression of the junction of the white and red skin inferoanterior to the 1st metatarsophalangeal joint.

Indications: Abdominal fullness, diarrhea, stomachache, edema of limbs, apoplexy, vomiting, constipation, absence of sweating in febrile diseases, heaviness of body with bone pain and infantile convulsion.

③ Taibai (Shu-Stream and Yuan-Primary point)

Location: In the medial border of the foot, in the depression posteroinferior to the 1st metatarsophalangeal joint, at the junction of the white and red skin.

Indications: Headache, stomachache, abdominal fullness, edema, dysentery, acute gastroenteritis, constipation, hemorrhoid, neuralgia and paralysis in the lower limbs.

④ Gongsun (Luo-Connecting point, one of the eight confluential points, communicating with Chong Channel)

Location: In the medial border of foot, anteroinferior to the base of the 1st metatarsal bone.

Indications: Stomachache, acute or chronic enteritis, vomiting, endometritis, irregular menstruation, and diseases of the reproductive system and the urinary system.

⑤ Shangqiu (Jing-Well point)

Location: In the depression anteroinferior to the medial malleolus, at the midpoint of the line connecting the tuberosity of navicular bone and the tip of the medial malleolus.

Indications: Gastritis, enteritis, indigestion, beriberi, edema, diseases of the ankle joint and its adjacent soft tissues, jaundice, infantile convulsion and hysteria.

⑥ Sanyinjiao (the confluential point of the Spleen, Liver and Kidney Channels)

Location: 3 cun above the medial malleolus, on the posterior border of tibia.

Indications: Borborygmus, abdominal fullness, loose stools, indigestion, irregular menstruation, metrostaxis and metrorrhagia, leukorrhagia, amenorrhea, prolapse of uterus, inflammation of pelvic cavity, impotence, emission, prostatitis, dysuria, enuresis, hernia, flaccidity of foot, insomnia, dizziness, neurosis, hypertension, urticaria, eczema, etc.

⑦ Diji (Xi-Cleft point)

Location: 3 cun below Yinlingquan.

Indications: Abdominal fullness, poor appetite, edema, diarrhea, dysuria, irregular menstruation, dysmenorrhea, hemorrhoid, emission, metrostaxis and metrorrhagia.

⑧ Yinlingquan (He-Sea point)

Location: In the depression inferior to the medial border of the epicondyle of the tibia.

Indications: Abdominal fullness, abdominal pain, edema, jaundice, vomiting, diarrhea, retention of urine, hernia, hypertension, emission, pain of knee, and damage of the soft tissues adjacent to the knee joint.

⑨ Xuehai

Location: 2 cun above the medial and superior margin of the patella.

Indications: Irregular menstruation, dysmenorrhea, hematuria, hypertension, various kinds of skin diseases such as eczema and urticaria, and diseases of the medial side of the knee joint.

(7) Extra and special points in the foot region (Fig. 19)

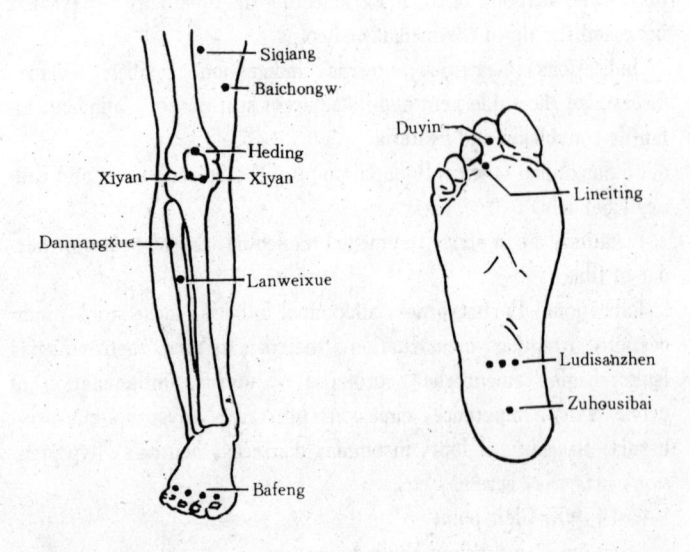

Fig. 19

① Dannangxue

Location: At the painful point about 2 cun below Yanglingquan.

Indications: Cholecystitis, cholelithiasis, biliary colic, biliary ascariasis.

② Lanweixue

Location: At the painful point about 2 cun below Zusanli.

Indications: Acute or chronic appendicitis.

③ Bafeng

Location: On the dorsum of foot, between the 1st and the 5th toes, at the junction of the white and red skin posterior to the web margin, 4 points on either side, 8 points in all.

Actions: Beriberi, swelling and pain of the dorsum of foot, pain and numbness of toes, headache, toothache, irregular menstruation, congestion of lung, malaria, snake bite, etc.

④ Qiduan

Location: At the tips of the toes, 0.1 cun away from the free border of the nail, 10 points in all.

Indications: Apoplexy, numbness of toes, swelling and pain of dorsum of foot and pain of foot.

⑤ Neihuaijian

Location: In the medial side of foot, at the prominence of the medial malleolus.

Indications: Pain in the lower teeth, sore throat, systremma in the medial side of foot and infantile aphasis.

⑥ Waihuaijian

Location: In the lateral side of foot, at the prominence of the external malleolus.

Indications: Systremma in the lateral side of foot, fever, chills, beriberi, convulsion of the toes, toothache and gonorrhea.

⑦ Duyin

Location: In the sole, at the midpoint of the distal metatarsal joint of the 2nd toe.

Indications: Sudden precardial pain, pain in the hypochondrium, vomiting, hematemesis, dead fetus, irregular menstruation, hernia, etc.

⑧ Lineiting

Location: In the sole, between the 2nd and 3rd metatarsal bones, opposite to Neiting.

Indications: Pain of toes, infantile convulsion, epilepsy and acute stomachache.

⑨ Zuzhongchong

Location: At the tip of the belly of the 3rd toe.

Indications: Cardiac failure, headache and epilepsy.

⑩ Yejing

Location: At the lateral end of the transverse crease of the distal segment of the little toe.

Indications: Night blindness, enuresis and swelling and redness of eyes.

⑪ Shimian

Location: At the center of the heel region.

Indications: Insomnia.

⑫ Niuxi

Location: Above the heel, at the midpoint of the junction of red and white skin.

Indications: Swelling and diabrosis of gums, palpitation, epistaxis, nasal obstruction, epilepsy, etc.

⑬ Ludisanzhen

Location: In the sole, 3 points in all, one of which is 1.5 cun anterior to the crossing point of the line connecting the midpoint of the line connecting the medial and external malleoluses and the heel and the midline of the sole, and the other two are 0.5 cun away from the point in the left and right respectively.

Indications: Headache, high fever, tinnitus, pain of the liver and spleen, stomachache, constipation, enteritis, dysentery, abdominal fluctuance, mastitis, ascites and hemiplegia.

⑭ Zuhousibai

Location: At the crossing point of the longitude midline of sole and the line drawing from the midpoint of the line connecting the tip of the external malleolus and the heel.

Indications: Headache, cerebrospinal menginitis, infantile convulsion, infantile vomiting, noctural urine, hemiplegia, prolapse of rectum and drops of foot.

⑮ Quanshengzu

Location: At the midpoint of the heel, in the midpoint of the transverse crease in the upper margin of the calcaneus.

Indications: Distocia, lumbago and esophageal convulsion.

4. The reflecting zones of foot

All the tissues and organs have their corresponding reflecting zones on the feet, or the nerve endings. When these nerve endings are massaged, the impulse produced will be transmitted to the neuroganglion of the spine at a speed of 60~120 meters/second, and then further sent to the related organs through the afferent nerve to regulate the function of the organs. Meanwhile, stimulation of the foot can improve blood circulation in the foot, increase filling of the tissues and help eliminate the metabolic products out of the body through the discharging system. So it can promote flow of Qi and Blood and regulate the functions of the Zang-Fu organs.

According to locations, the foot reflecting zones can be divided into four groups, the reflecting zones on the sole of foot, the reflecting zones on the medial side of the foot, the reflecting zones on the lateral side of the foot and the reflecting zones on the dorsum of foot.

Massage on pathological reflecting zones on both feet can treat diseases of all the systems, including the circulatory system, the respiratory system, the digestive system, the urinary system, the reproductive system, the skeleton system, the five sense organs (the eye, the ear, the nose, the mouth and the throat) and the endocrine system.

The reflecting zones in the sole of the foot include these on the right foot and these on the left foot.

(1) The reflecting zones of the right foot (Fig. 20)
(2) The reflecting zones of the left foot (Fig. 21)
(3) The reflecting zones of the lateral side of foot (Fig. 22)
(4) The reflecting zones of the medial side of foot (Fig. 23)
(5) The reflecting zones on the dorsum of foot (Fig. 24)

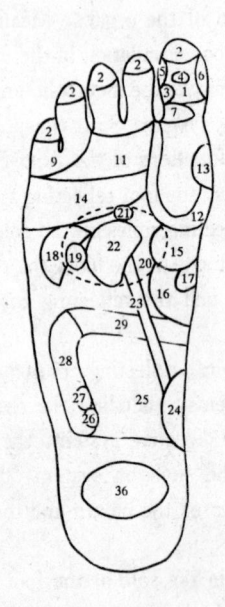

Fig. 20

1. Cerebrum (the left hemisphere)
2. Frontal Sinus (the left hemisphere)
3. Brain Stem, Cerebellum
4. Pituitary Gland
5. Temporal Lobe and Trigerminal Nerve (the left)
6. Nose
7. Neck
8. Eye (the left)
9. Ear (the left)
11. Trapezius Muscle (the Neck and Shoulder) (the right)
12. Thyriod Gland
13. Accessory Thyroid Gland
14. Bronchus and Lung (the right)
15. Stomach
16. Duodenum, Liver
17. Pancreas
18. Liver
19. Gallbladder
20. Celliac Plexus (the digestive system)
21. Adrenal Gland (the right)
22. Kidney (the right)
23. Ureter (the right)
24. Bladder
25. Small Intestine
26. Ileocum and Appendix
27. Ileocecal Valve
28. Ascending Colon
29. Transverse Colon
36. Genital Gland (ovary or testis) (the right)

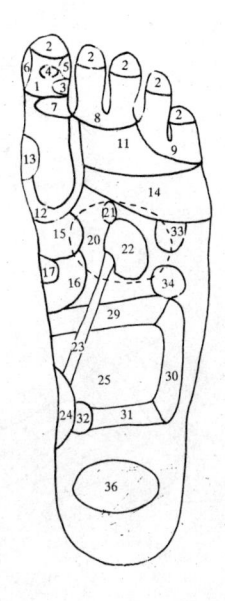

Fig. 21

1. Cerebrum (the right hemisphere)
2. Frontal Sinus (the right hemisphere)
3. Brain Stem, Cerebellum
4. Pituitary Gland
5. Temporal Lobe and Trigerminal Nerve (the left)
6. Nose
7. Neck
8. Eye (the right)
9. Ear (the right)
11. Trapezius Muscle (the Neck and Shoulder) (the left)
12. Thyriod Gland
13. Accessory Thyroid Gland
14. Bronchus and Lung (the right)
15. Stomach
16. Duodenum
17. Pancreas
20. Celliac Plexus (the digestive system)
21. Adrenal Gland (the left)
22. Kidney (the left)
23. Ureter (the left)
24. Bladder
25. Small Intestine
29. Transverse Colon
30. Descending Colon
31. Rectum
32. Anus
33. Heart
34. Spleen
36. Genital Gland (ovary or testis) (the left)

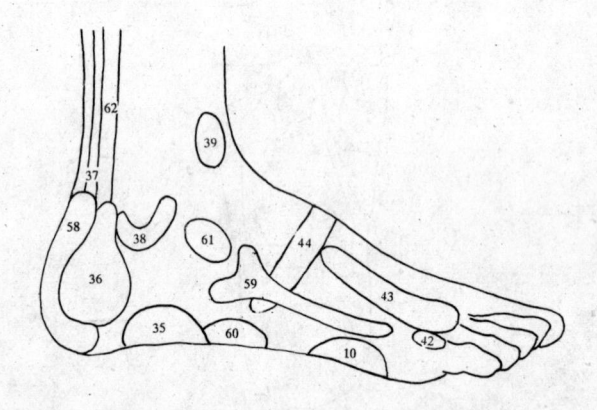

Fig. 22

10. Shoulder
35. Knee
36. Genital Glands (Ovary, Salpinx or Testis)
37. Systremma
38. Hip Joint
39. Lymph Gland of Upper Body
42. Equilibrium Organs
44. Chest (Breast)
58. Outer Coccyx
59. Scapula
60. Elbow Joint
61. Rib
62. Sciatic Nerve

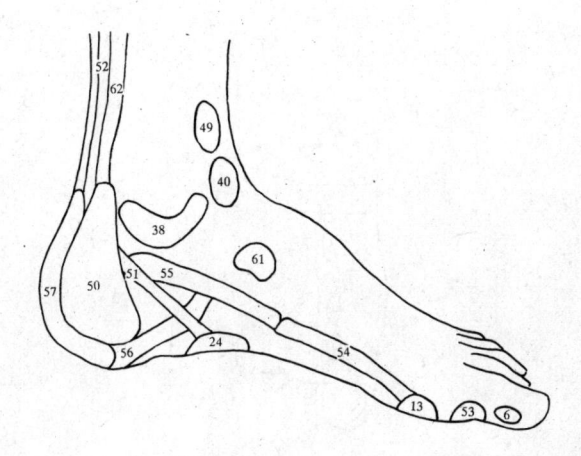

Fig. 23

6. Nose
13. Accessory Thyroid Gland
24. Bladder
38. Hip Joint
40. Lymph Gland of Lower Body
49. Inguinal Groove
50. Uterus (Postrate Gland)
51. Penis and Vagina (Urethra)
52. Anus (hemorrhoid) and Rectum
53. Cervical Vertebrae
54. Thoracic Vertebrae
55. Lumbar Vertebrae
56. Sacral Vertebrae and Coccyx
57. Inner Coccyx

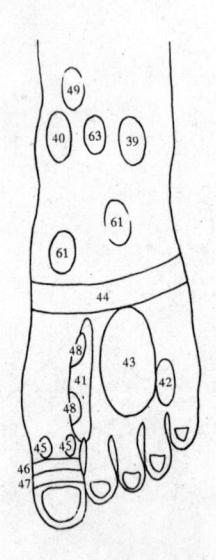

Fig. 24

39. Lymph Nodes of the Upper Body
40. Lymph Nodes of the Lower Body
41. Thoracic Lymph Gland
42. Equilibrium Organ
43. Chest (Breast)
44. Diaphragm
45. Tonsil
46. Lower Palate
47. Upper Palate
48. Throat and Bronchus
49. Inguinal Groove
61. Rib
63. Jiexi (Phlegm Dissolvement)

5. Brief introduction to each of the reflecting zones
(1) The reflecting zones of the right sole
① Cerebrum (the left hemisphere)

Location: In the belly of the great toe. The left and the right cerebrum hemispheres are reflected crossly in the soles of the feet. That is, the pathological reflecting zone of the right cerebrum hemisphere is in the sole of the left foot, while that of the right is in the sole of the right foot.

Manipulation: Push-press the zone from the tip of the great toe to the heel with the thumb for 5 minutes.

Indications: Hypertension, cerebrovascular diseases, concussion of brain, dizziness, headache, insomnia, central paralysis, optic damage, etc.

② Brain Stem and Cerebellum

Location: In the sole, at the root of the great toe distal to the first metatarsophangeal bone. The left and the right cerebrum are reflected crossly.

Indications: Brain tumors, concussion of brain, hypertension, hypotension, insomnia, headache, damage of soft tissues, etc.

Manipulation: Finger-pressing or twisting manipulation at a fixed point for 5 minutes.

③ Pituitary Gland

Location: At the center of the belly of the great toe, at the depth of the reflecting zone of the Cerebrum.

Indications: All the disturbance of the endocrine system.

Manipulation: Press and knead deeply at a fixed point for $3 \sim 5$ minutes.

④ Frontal Sinus

Location: At the tips of the toes, 10 in number. The left and the right frontal sinuses are reflected crossly in feet. That is, the left frontal sinus is reflected on the right foot, and the right frontal sinus is on the left foot.

Indications: Cerebrovascular diseases, concussion of brain, headache, dizziness, insomnia, diseases of the eyes, the ears, the nose and the mouth.

Manipulation: Press and knead the tips of the toes one by one for 5 minutes.

⑤ Temporal Lobe

Location: At an angle of 45 degree on the lateral corner of the belly of the great toe. The bilateral trigerminal nerves and the frontal lobes are reflected crossly on the two feet. That is, the reflecting zone of the left trigerminal nerve and temporal lobe is on the right foot, while that of the right is on the left foot.

Indications: Paralysis of the facial nerve, migraine, mumps, diseases of the ear, nasopharyngeal cancer, insomnia, spasm of the facial muscle and facial neuralgia.

Manipulation: Press with finger pressing method at a fixed point for 5 minutes.

⑥ Eyes

Location: At the root of the second and third toes in the sole. The two eyes are reflected in the sole crossly. Or, the left eye is reflected in the right foot and the right eye is in the left foot.

Indications: Optic neuritis, conjunctivitis, keratitis, myopia, farsightedness, vertigo, cataract, eyeground bleeding, photophobia, lacrmation, etc.

Manipulation: Press with a flexed finger at a fixed point for 5 minutes.

⑦ Ear

Location: At the root of the fourth and the fifth toes in the sole. The two ears are reflected corssly in the soles of the feet. Or, the Ear in the right foot should be treated when the left ear has diseases, and the Ear in the left should be treated when the right ear has diseases.

Indications: Various kinds of ear diseases such as otitis media, tinnitus, subaural lymphatitis, and nasopharyngeal cancer.

Manipulation: Press or knead with finger at a fixed point for 5 minutes.

⑧ Nose

Location: At an angle about 45 degree at the base of the belly of the first phalanx of the great toe. It is reflected in the feet crossly.

Or, the left nose is reflected in the right foot and the right nose in the left foot.

Indictaions: Acute or chronic rhinitis, allergic rhinitis, nasal sinusitis, epistaxis and infection of the upper respiratory tract.

Manipulation: Press at a fixed area for 5 minutes.

⑨ Neck

Location: In the second phalanx medial to the great toe, in the sole of both feet, behind the first phalanx. The reflecting zones of the bilateral necks are all in the same sides of the feet.

Indications: Soreness of the neck and nape, rigidity of the neck, spondylopathy of the neck, cervical hyperosteogeny, hypertension, neck stiffness, etc.

Manipulation: Press with one finger from th tip of the great toe to the root of the toe for 3~5 minutes.

⑩Thyroid Gland

Location: In the sole of the feet, at the root of the great toe.

Indications: Thyroiditis, thyroid hypertrophy, hyperthyroidism, palpitation, insomnia and over weight.

Manipulation: Press with the thumb from the heel to the toes for 3 minutes.

⑪Accessory Thyroid Gland

Location: In the medial border of sole, at the junction of the 1st metatarsal bone and the 1st phalangeal bone. The reflecting zones of the accessory thyroid glands are on the same sides of the feet.

Indications: Hypoparathyroidism, hyperparathyroidism, allergic reaction, soreness of tendons and muscles, numberness and convulsion of the limbs, weakness of the nails, nausea, vomiting, etc.

Manipulation: Press digitally at a fixed position for 3 minutes.

⑫Shoulder

Location: On the lateral sides of the palmar side of the feet, at the prominent metatarsal joint on the lateral border of the little toe. The reflecting zones of the left shoulder and these of the right shoulder are on the same side, or the left shoulder is in the left foot and the right shoulder is in the right foot.

Indications: Periarthritis of shoulder, neck-shoulder syndrome, numbness and weakness of the upper limbs, damage of the soft tissues adjacent to the shoulder joint, and habitual dislocation of shoulder joint.

Manipulation: Press digitally at a fixed position for 3 minutes.

⑬ Trapezius Muscle

Location: Inferior to the Ear and Eye in the sole, being a transverse belt-like zone from the 1st metatarsal bone to the lateral side of the foot. The left and right trapezius muscles are in the same side of the feet.

Indications: Soreness and pain of the neck and shoulder, weakness and numbness of hands and difficulty of the shoulder joint in movement.

Manipulation: Press with thumb from the medial side to the lateral side for 5 minutes.

⑭ Esophagus

Location: Situated between the 1st metatarsal bone and the 5th metatarsal bone, taking a shape of a cone or strip.

Indications: Various kinds of esophageal diseases.

Manipulation: Push and press from the toes towards the heel for about 3 minutes.

⑮ Stomach

Location: In the middle and lower part of the 1st metatarsal bone of the soles.

Indications: Stomachache, excessive gastric acid, gastric ulcer, acute or chronic gastritis, indigestion, gastroptosis, etc.

Manipulation: Push and press from the toes to the heel for about 5 minutes.

⑯ Duodenum

Location: At the base of the 1st metatarsal bone of feet, posterior to Stomach.

Indications: Diseases of the stomach and the duodenum, indigestion, abdominal fullness and distension, duodenal ulcer, etc.

Manipulation: Push from the toes toward the heel for 5 minutes.

⑰ Liver

Location: Between the 4th and the 5th metatarsl bones of the right sole, below the Lung. This reflecting zone only exists in the right sole.

Indications: Hepatitis, cirrhosis of liver, malnutrition and fatigue caused by dysfunctional or poor liver function.

Manipulation: Press or knead with fingers from the toes towards the heel for 5 minutes.

⑱ Gallbladder

Location: Between the 3rd and the 4th metatarsal bones of the right sole, below the Lung and within the Liver. This is a reflecting zone seen only in the left sole.

Indications: Cholelithiasis, cholecystitis, hepatitis, jaundice and indigestion.

Manipulation: Press or knead with fingers at the fixed spot for 5 minutes.

⑲ Pancreas

Location: In the middle and lower portions of the 1st metatarsal bones of the soles, like a hycinth bean in shape, between the Stomach and the Duodenum.

Indications: Diabetes, pancreatitis, and other diseases of the metabolic system.

Manipulation: Push with the finger flexed from the toes towards the heel for 5 minutes.

⑳ Trachea and Lung

Location: Below the Trapezius muscle of the soles, running from the Thyroid Gland to Shoulder in the lateral side of the sole, being strip like in shape. The Lung is in the sole of the same side, or the reflecting zones of the right lung and trachea are on the right side, while the left Lung is in the left side.

Indications: Pneumonia, emphysema, tuberculosis of the lung, bronchitis, chest stuffiness, asthma, etc.

Manipulation: Push with the thumb from the medial side to the lateral side of 5 minutes.

㉑ Small Intestine

Location: In the depression from the metatarsal bones and cuneiform bone to the heel, surrounded by the reflecting zones of the ascending colon, transverse colon and the descending colon.

Indications: Abdominal fluctuance, diarrhea, abdominal pain, acute or chronic gastroenteritis, etc.

Manipulation: Push with fingers along the distribution of the colon for 3~5 minutes.

㉒ Large Intestine

Location: In the centers of the soles, distributing transversely across the soles, taking a shape of a strip paralling to the lateral borders of the feet, and corresponding to the region from the space of the 4th and 5th metatarsal bones to the calceus. In the right sole, it serves as the reflecting zone of the cecum, appendix, ileocolic valve, ascending colon and transverse colon.

Indications: Constipation, abdominal pain, diarrhea, distension in the upper abdomen, appendicitis, enteritis, hemorrhoids, etc.

Manipulation: Push with finger-pressing method along the distribution of colon for 3~5 minutes.

㉓ Kidney

Location: In the depression a bit posterior to the "∧" shaped grooves of the soles.

Indications: Kidney stone, stone of the ureter, renal insufficiency, hypertension, atherosclerosis, varicosis of veins, uremia, migratory kidney, renal hydronephrosis, oliguria, edema, rheumatic fever, arthritis, eczema, etc.

Manipulation: Press and knead with finger at fixed spots for 5 minutes.

㉔ Adrenal Gland

Location: In the depession below the top of the "∧" shaped groove in the soles.

Indications: Kidney stone, disorders of the kidney, arrhythmia, faint, asthma, atheroscelerosis, hypertension, rheumatic fever, arthritis, uremia, allergic diseases, chronic insufficiency of the paraadrenal gland, etc.

Manipulation: Push and press at a fixed spot for 3 minutes.

㉕ Ureter

Location: In the strip zone distributing from the Kidney to the

Bladder of the soles.

Indications: Stone of the kidney, ureter and bladder, hydronephrosis caused by stenosis of the ureter, cystitis, hypertension, atherosclerosis, rheumatic fever, arthritis, retention of urine, etc.

Manipulation: Push with the thumb the strip-like zone of Ureter from the Kidney toward the Bladder for 5 minutes.

㉖ Bladder

Location: Lateral to the abductor muscle of the great toe, below the nut bone in the medial side of the sole.

Indications: Stone of stomach, urethra and bladder, infection of the urinary system, diseases of bladder, hypertension, atherosclerosis, etc.

Manipulation: Push, or press and knead at a fixed point for 5 minutes.

㉗ Congenital Gland (Testis or Ovary)

Location: In the centre of the calcaneus of soles.

Indications: Hyposexualism, sterility, bloody leukorrhea, abdominal pain during ovulation, menstrual tension syndrome, etc.

㉘ Celliac Plexus

Location: In the centre of the soles, adjacent to the Kidney and the Stomach.

Indications: Abdominal fullness, diarrhea, and gastrointestinal neurosism marked by nervousness, irritability and abdominal distension.

Manipulation: Push and press around the reflecting zone from the upper to the lower for 5 minutes.

㉙ Buttock

Location: On the lateral border of the cancaneus of the soles.

Indications: Inflammation of the hip, pain of the hip joint, sciatica and damage of the coccygeal bone.

Manipulation: Press digitally at a fixed site for 3 minutes.

㉚ Sciatic Nerve

Location: Located at the posterior border of the cancaneus of the soles, taking a shape of a horseshoe.

Indications: Sciatica, inflammation of the sciatic nerve and injury of the sciatic nerve.

Manipulation: Push with the thumb along the border of the heel from the medial border to the lateral border for 3 minutes.

㉛ Jiangxueyadian

Location: On the lower border of the Cerebellum of the great toe, lateral to the Neck.

Indications: Hypertension, cerebroartherosclerosis, etc.

Manipulation: Press at a fixed point for 3 minutes.

㉜ Pelvic Cavity

Location: Above the heels of the soles, on the upper border of the Genital Gland.

Indications: Insomnia and neurosism of various types.

Manipulation: Press at a fixed position for 3 minutes.

The above mentioned are the reflecting zones in the right sole, of which the cecum, ileocecal valve and the transverse colon are only seen in the right sole. Besides, the reflecting zones of heart and spleen are absent in the right sole.

(2) The reflecting zones of the left sole

Most of the reflecting zones of the left sole are the same with those in the right sole, but the reflecting zones of the liver and gallbladder are absent in the left sole. Besides, the reflecting zone of the large intestine in the left sole is different from that in the righ because it is composed of the transverse colon, the descending colon and the anus. The following is an introduction to the pathologic reflecting zones specific to the left sole, which include the reflecting zones of the heart and the spleen.

① Heart (Left sole, 17)

Location: Between the 4th and the 5th metatarsal bones in the left sole, below the Lung.

Indications: Angina pectoris, cardiac failure, arrhythmia, shock, cardiac defect, congenital or acquired cardiac diseases, etc.

Manipulation: Press and knead vertically with finger-kneading method for 3~5 minutes.

② Spleen (Left sole, 18)

Location: In a zone about one finger's breadth below the Heart in the left sole.

Indications: Anemia, poor appetite, indigestion, inflammation, common cold, skin diseases, and cancers related to dysfunction of the spleen.

Manipulation: Press vertically with finger-pressing method at a fixed position for 4 minutes.

(3) The reflecting zones in the lateral side of foot

① The Lower Abdomen

Location: In the groove posterior to the ankle in the lateral side of the foot, being a strip-like zone starting from the external malleolus to a point 3 cun above.

Indications: Abdominal pain, amenorrhea, dysmenorrhea, premenstrual tension syndrome, irregular menstrual cycles, injury of abdominal soft tissues, etc.

Manipulation: Push and press upward from the posterior zone of the ankle with finge-pressing method for 3 minutes.

② Hip Joint

Location: Located in the lateral side of the foot, in the zone below the external malleolus.

Indications: Pain of the hip joint and sciatica.

③ Congenital Gland (Ovary, fallopian tube or testis and accessory testis)

Location: In the lateral side of the foot, below the external malleolus, in a triangular zone posterior to the lateral side of the calceus.

Indications: Hyposexuality, sterility, testitis, accessory testitis, inflammation of the fallopian tube, dysmenorrhea, irregular menstruation, abdominal pain in the ovulatory stage, and menopausal syndrome.

Manipulation: Push and press with finger-pressing method at a fixed zone from the lower to the upper for 5 minutes.

④ Knee

Location: On the lateral arc of the foot, posterior to the tuberosity of the calceus, being a zone of half-moon shape.

Indications: Inflammation of the knee joint, traumatic injury of the soft tissues of the knee joint, pain of the knee joint, softening of the hip bone and injury of the menisus.

Manipulation: Press with finger-pressing method at a fixed position for 4 minutes.

⑤ Elbow Joint

Location: On the lateral arc of the foot, in the depression around the prominence of the 5th metatarsal bone, posterior to the reflecting zone of the knee joint.

Indications: Soreness and pain of the elbow joint, injury of soft tissues of the elbow joint, tennis elbow, etc.

Manipulation: Press with finger-pressing method at a fixed position for 5 minutes.

⑥ Shoulder

Location: On the lateral arc of the foot, in the depression posterior to the 5th metatarso-phalangeal articulation.

Indications: Periarthritis of shoulder, injury of the soft tissues around the shoulder, neck-shoulder syndrome, weakness or numbness of the upper limbs, etc.

Manipulation: Press and knead with finger at a fixed position for 4 minutes.

⑦ Scapula

Location: On the lateral side of the dorsum of foot, in a strip shaped zone formed by the 4th and 5th metatarsal bones and the cuboid bone.

Indications: Stiff neck, soreness of scapular region, periarthritis of shoulder, dysfunction of the shoulder joint, and injury of soft tissues of the shoulder, the back and the neck.

Manipulation: Press and push with thumb backwards from the toes for 5 minutes.

⑧ Tail Bone

Location: On the lateral side of the foot heel, being a strip-like zone distributing along the posterior zone of the tuberosity of the calceus.

Indications: Sciatica, injury of sacral vertebrae and its sequala.

Manipulation: Push and press anteriorly from the heel for 3 minutes.

⑨ Lymph Gland of the Upper Body

Location: Posterior to the external malleolus, in the depression between two small bones.

Indications: Inflammation, cysts, cancers, fever, decline of immunological function, cellulitis, etc.

Manipulation: Push and press at a fixed position for 3 minutes.

(4) The reflecting zones in the medial side of foot

① Cervical Vertebra

Location: In the medial side of the great toes, in an zone of 45° with the second phalangeal bone.

Indications: Rigidity, stiffness or aching of neck and nape.

Manipulation: Twist and rub for 3 minutes in the reflecting zone.

② Thoracic Vertebra

Location: In the medial border of the arch of the foot, from the inferior zone of the first metatarsal bone to the joint of the first cubitale.

Indications: Aching in the back, protrudence of the intervertebral disc of the thoracic vertebra, hyperplasia of the cervical vertebrae and other diseases of the thoracic vertebrae.

Manipulation: Push and press with finger-pressing method from the anterior part to the posterior part for 3 minutes.

③ Lumbar Vertebra

Location: In the medial border of the foot arc, from the cubitale to the inferior zone of the navicular bone.

Indications: Soreness and pain in the lumbar region, protrudence of the intervertebral discs, hyperplasia of the lumbar vertebra and other diseases of the lumbar vertebra.

Manipulation: Push and press with finger-pressing method from the anterior part to the posterior part for 3 minutes.

④ Sacral Vertebra

Location: In the medial border of the foot arc, connecting with the Lumbar Vertebra in its anterior part and the Tail Bone in its posterior part, distributed from the inferior zone of talcus to the calceus.

Indications: Hyperplasia of the calceus, traumatic injury of the sacral vertebra, sciatica, and diseases of the visceral organs in the pelvic cavity.

Manipulation: Push and press toward the heel from the toes for 3 minutes.

⑤ Inner Tail Bone

Location: In the medial border of the foot arch, posterior to calceus, being a strip shaped zone distributing posteriorly from the tuberosity of calceus.

Indications: Sciatica, sequala of injury of tail bone, etc.

Manipulation: Push and press with finger-pressing method anteriorly from the heel for 3 minutes.

⑥ Hip Joint

Location: In the inferior zone of the medial malleolus, being an arc-shaped zone.

Indications: Sciatica, injury of soft tissues of hip joint, pain or other diseases of the hip joint.

Manipulation: Push and press from the inferoanterior part to the posterosuperior part for 3 minutes.

⑦ Uterus (Prostate Gland) and Vagina (Urethra)

Location: In the medial side of the calceus. The zone extending backward from the reflecting zone of bladder to the zone between the talcus and navicular bone is the reflecting zone of urethra or vagina; while that going upward obliquely to the inferior zone of the malleolus is the reflecting zone of uterus or prostate gland.

Indications: Male (Prostate Gland): Hyperplasia of prostate gland marked by frequent urine, hematuria and oligura. Female: Dysmenorrhea, maldevelopment of uterus and other diseases of the uterus. Urethra: urethritis marked by pain in the urethra.

Manipulation: Push and press from the lower to the upper for 5 minutes.

⑧ Rectum and Anus

Location: In the groove posterior to the medial malleolus, having a length of 4 fingers breadth, distributed upwards from the tip of the medial malleolus.

Indications: Rectal inflammation, constipation, hemorrhoids, anal fissure, and varicosis of vein.

Manipulation: Push and press with finger-pressing method superiorly from the posterior aspect of the calceus.

⑨ Inguinal Groove

Location: One cun above the tip of the medial malleolus, being an zone formed in the medial aspect of the tibia.

Indications: Diseases of the reproductive system, sexual disability, etc.

Manipulation: Press and push with finger-pressing method from the upper to the lower for 5 minutes.

(5) The reflecting zones on the dorsum of foot

① Lymph Gland of the Upper Body

Location: On the dorsum of foot, anterior to the external malleolus, in the depression formed by the talcus and the navicular bone.

Indications: Inflammation of various kinds, fever, decline of immunological function, cellulitis, cyst, cancer, etc.

Manipulation: Press or knead with finger at a fixed position for 3 minutes.

② Lymph Gland of the Lower Body

Location: On the dorsum of foot, anterior to the medial malleolus, in the depression formed by the talcus and the navicular bone.

Indications: Inflammation, edema of leg, swelling of ankle, cyst, fever, decline of immunological function, cancers, cellulitis, etc.

Manipulation: Press or knead with fingers from the upper part to the lower part for 3 minutes.

③ Diaphragm

Location: In the strip like zone formed by the metatarsal bone and the cubitale, distributing across the left and right sides of the dorsum.

Indications: Hiccup, abdominal fullness, abdominal pain, nausea, vomiting, etc.

Manipulation: Press and push from the midpoint of the reflecting zone to its bilateral sides for 3 minutes.

④ Lymph Gland of the Chest

Location: In the space between the first and the second metatarsal bones on the dorsum of foot.

Indications: Inflammation, cancer, tumor, fever, cysts, breast masses and deficiency of antibodies.

Manipulation: Push and press with finger-pressing method from the toes to the heel for 3 minutes.

⑤ Liver Meridian Gland

Location: On the dorsum of foot, in the space formed by the first and the second metatarsal bones, posterior to the reflecting zone of lymph gland of the chest.

Indications: Used as a supplementary for treatment of liver diseases.

Manipulation: Press and knead with finger-pressing method for 3 minutes.

⑥ Chest

Location: On the dorsum of foot, in the zone formed by the second, third and fourth metatarsal bones.

Indications: Chest stuffiness, asthma, mastitis, carcinoma of mammary gland, breast congestion or swelling before menstruation, cysts and injury of the soft tissues in the chest.

Manipulation: Push with thumb from the anterior part to the posterior part for 5 minutes.

⑦ Larynx and Trachea

Location: In the articulation of the first and second metatarsal bones on the dorsum of foot, posterior to the Lymph Gland of the Chest.

Indications: Sore throat, cough, asthma, bronchitis, common cold, laryngitis, and feeble voice.

Manipulation: Push and press with finger-pressing method towards the toes from the heel for 5 minutes.

⑧ Inner Ear (Balancing organ)

Location: In the region of the 4th and the 5th metatarsal bones on the dorsum of foot.

Indications: Dizziness, hypertension, vertigo, hypotension, balance disturbance, car-sickness, boat-sickness, tinnites and decline of the function of the inner ear.

Manipulation: Press and knead with finger-pressing method anteriorly from the heel for 5 minutes.

⑨ Tonsil

Location: On the doral aspect of the great toe, in the bilateral sides of the 2nd metatarsal bone.

Indications: Common cold, swelling, pain or enlargement of tonsil, pyogenic tonsilitis and the headache caused by it.

Manipulation: Press and push with finger-pressing method at a fixed position for 5 minutes.

⑩ The Upper Palate and the Lower Palate

Location: In the two strip-like zones superior and inferior to the transverse crease of the interphalangeal articulation of the great toe, which correspond to the upper palate and the lower palate respectively.

Indications: Aphtha, toothache, snoring, inflammation of the upper or the lower palate.

Manipulation: Twist the reflecting zone with thumb for 5 minutes.

⑪ Lymph Gland of the Whole Body

Location: In the creases of the toes of foot and in the upper border of Tonsil in the great toe.

Indications: Inflammation of the whole body and decline of the immunological function.

Manipulation: Point and press toe by toe, 2 minutes for each toe.

Treatment of Diseases with Foot Point-Zone Massage Therapy

*F*oot massage theapy is an effective method that is widely applied in treatment of diseases of various departments in the clinic. It can be used as both a health care technique and a therapeutic method. It can relieve symptoms, improve the patients' general conditions, promote metabolism and directly cure diseases. Therefore, it is not only effective for diseases of the internal medicine, but also effective for surgical diseases, gynecological diseases, pediatric diseases and dermatological diseases.

Diseases of the Internal Medicine

Angina Pectoris

This is a syndrome caused by temporary and sudden ischemia and hypoxia of the cardiac muscles. Coronary atherosclerosis serves as the main causative factor, and other cardiac diseases such as the vular diseases, syphilitic aortitis complicated by stenosis of the opening of the coronary artery, hypertrophic cardiomyopathy, anemia and hyperthyroidism can also lead to attack of the disease.

Essentials of Diagnosis
Clinicl manifestations:

1. Remarkable induction factors, such as fatigue, excitation and overeat.

2. Sudden presence of oppressed pain in the retrosternal or precardic region, which radiates to the left shoulder and arm and lasts 1 ~5 minutes.

3. The condition can be relieved by rest or administration of nitroglycerin.

Supplementary examinations
When the disease attacks, ischemic ST-T segment changes can be found, and when the attack stops, the ECG load test may be positive.

Massage treatment
1. Prescription of foot points: Knead with the border of nail bilateral Shuiquan, Yongquan and the bilateral Duyin, press and knead bilateral Taichong and Taixi.

2. Prescription of the reflecting zones: Press and knead the Heart of the left foot at selected points, and push and press the Adrenal Glands, Kidney, Ureter and Bladder on the two feet. Then, hold and twist the toes, and rub heavily the midline in the sole.

Remarks
1. The above prescribed groups of points are to be treated twice a day. The Heart should be pressed gently for a short time.

2. This therapy is effective for angina pectoris. Constant use of the therapy can reduce the attacks and relieve symptoms of the angina pectoris.

3. If this therapy is administered in the attack stage of the disease, it can relieve the symptom as a supplementary treatment. However, if patient is experiencing a persistent sharp pain or even presents cold sweating and fails to response to the massage therapy, rest and administration of nitroglycerin, it suggests cardiac infarct, and comprehensive treatments should be given at once.

Atherosclerosis

Usually this term denotes non-inflammatory, degenerative and hypertrophic lesion of the artery which will finally lead to thickening and hardening of the arterial wall and narrowing of the lumen of the artery. This disease consists of three patterns: Atheriosclerosis, medial calcification of artery and the sclerosis of the small or fine artery. Mostly, the first is referred to as the atherosclerosis.

This disease usually involves the major or middle-sized arteries, causing such severe results as obstruction of the artery or bleeding due to rupture of the arterial wall. The aorta, coronary artery and cerebral artery are the most often affected.

Essentials of Diagnosis

General manifestations:

1. The physical strength declines, and the superficial arteries are found to be widened, hardened and prolonged.

2. Sclerosis of the coronary artery, which is marked by elevation of the systolic pressure, increase of the difference of the systolic and the diastolic pressure, strengthening of the second heart sound in the aortic zone, and systolic murmur.

3. Sclerosis of the coronary artery, which often results in angina pectoris and cardiac infarct.

4. Sclerosis of the cerebral artery, which often gives rise to dizziness, headache, syncope, cerebrovascular accidents, dementia due to encephalatrophy, psychopathy, etc.

Supplementary examination:

Elevation of blood cholesterol and triglyceride, abnormality of lipoprotein electrophoresis, dilation and calcinosis of aorta on X-ray examination.

Massage treatment

1. Prescription of foot points: Press and knead bilateral Zusanli and Sanyinjiao; point and knead bilateral Taichong and Xiaxi; and rub bilateral Yongquan.

2. Prescription of the foot reflecting zones: Point and knead bilateral Adrenal Gland, push and press Kidney, Ureter and Bladder of the bilateral feet and the left Heart and Spleen.

Remarks

1. The above points or zones are to be treated once in the daytime and once before sleep everyday.

2. Constant use of this treatment can soften vessels, dredge the Heart vessels and prevent and treat atherosclerosis.

Hypertension

Hypertension can be divided into the primary hypertension and the secondary hypertension. The former refers to a disease with elevation of blood pressure as its main clinical manifestation with unknown causes, or the hypertensive diseases.

Essentials of Diagnosis

1. Criteria of diagnosis: According to suggestion of the World Health Organization, hypertension is indicated if an adult has a systolic pressure of 21.3 kPa or a sytolic pressure of 12.7 kPa.

2. Clinical manifetstations: According to the clinical manifestations, this disease can be classified as the progressive type and the accelerated type.

Progressive hypertension: This type has a slow progress. It is marked by headache, insomnia and forgetfulness initially and organic damage of the heart, brain and kidney, elevation of blood pressure, hypertrophy of the heart with murmur, disorders of the optic fundus and decline of the kidney function in its later stage.

Accelerated hypertension: This type is characterized by remarkable elevation of blood pressure, a diastolic pressure constantly higher than 17.3 kPa, severe damage of the brain, the heart and the kidney, eyeground bleeding and exudation, edema of optic disc, with a tendency to develop acute cerebrovascular diseases, cardiac failure and uremia.

3. Classfications of stages of hypertension

The 1st stage: Hypertension without symptoms of the heart, brain and kidney damage.

The 2nd stage: Hypertension with one of the following signs: Hypertrophy of the left ventricle found on physical examination, X-ray examination, electrocardiograph or echocardiogram; stricture of arteries in eyeground; proteinuria or increase of the creatinine concentration of plasma.

The 3rd stage: Hypertension with one of the following signs: Cerebral hemorrhage or hypertensive encephalopathy; cardiac failure; renal failure, bleeding of eyeground or edema of optic disc.

Massage treatment

1. Prescription of foot points: Press and knead bilateral Zusanli, Weizhong, Ququan, Sanyinjiao, Taichong and Taixi; point and press Jiangxueyadian of the two feet; and rub the bilateral Yongquan until a hot sensation is felt by patient.

2. Prescription of the reflecting zones: Point and press bilateral Adrenal Gland in the soles, then push and press the Kidney, Ureter and Bladder in the soles of the two feet; and push and press the Cerebrum, Cerebellum and the Pituitary Glands in the soles of the two feet.

3. Shake and tract toes of the feet, rub the sole, massage the heel and push the zone between the first and the second metatarsal bones on the dorsum.

Remarks

1. The above points and zones are to be treated twice a day.

2. Constant use of the treatment can prevent and treat hypertension and has a good therapeutic or rehabilitating effect on progressive hypertension or the hypertension in the 1st and the 2nd stages; and can be used as a supplementary treatment for the accelerated type of the hypertension in the 3rd stage.

3. Patients should avoid emotional stimuli, live a regular life, and do appropriate physical exercises. Greasy and fatty food and strong alcohol should be restricted.

Hypotension

Hypotension is of two types, the acute and the chronic. It is caused by neurosis, vegetative nerve functional disturbance, functional disturbance of the endocrine system, chronic consumptive diseases, malnutrition, cardiovascular diseases and drug reactions.

Essentials of Diagnosis

1. In the clinic, a blood pressure with a systolic pressure of 12 kPa and a diastolic pressure of 8 kPa is called hypotension.

2. Clinical Manifestations: Patients often have such accompanying manifestations as dizziness, tinnitus, palpitation, vertigo, polyhidrosis, pale, cold limbs, weakness, or even nausea, vomiting, syncope and shock.

Massage treatment

1. Prescription of foot points: Press and knead bilateral Zusanli and Sanyinjiao; point and press bilateral Taichong and Neiting; press with the nail and knead Zhongchong and Zulinqi; and point, knead and then rub the bilateral Yongquan; hold and twist the third toe.

2. Prescription of the foot reflecting zones: Point and knead the Heart in the sole, the heel and the medial and external malleoluses; then, push and press Kidney, Ureter and Bladder in the bilateral soles; hold, twist and knead Cerebrum of the feet; knead and twist Labyrinth on the dorsums of the feet and the Genital Glands in the soles.

Remarks

1. The above points and zones are to be treated twice a day.

2. The manipulation should be a little deep and heavy for treatment of acute hypotension to produce a remarkable soreness and distending feeling. It should be gentle and soft and lasts a longer time when used for keep health to produce a discomfort effect. Constant application of the massage can improve the function of the circulatory system.

Sinus Tachycardia

This refers to a condition marked by a frequence of the impulse sent off from the sinus being over 100 times per minutes in adult.

Essential of Diagnosis

1. Patient has a discomfortable feeling due to acceleration of the heart beats, palpitation and shortness of breath. The heart rate in adult is over 100 beats per minutes, but rarely it is over 150 beats per minutes.

2. It is mainly related to the hypovagotonia and sympathetic excitation and is often induced by fatigue, emotional excitment, intake of alcohol and strong tea.

3. On ECG examination, there is sinus P wave, an PP interval shorter than 0.6 sec. and a PR interval longer than 0.12 sec. The P wave may overlap the previous T wave.

Massage Treatment

1. Prescription of the foot points: Press and knead bilateral Sanyinjiao; point and knead bilateral Taichong and Zhaohai; press the nail and knead Shimian points on the heels, twist the second and the third toes of the feet from the roots to the tips of the toes for 3 or 5 times, and knead with finger and then rub Yongquan with palm.

2. Prescription of the foot reflecting zones: Point and press the Adrenal Glands in the soles of feet, push horinzontally Thyroid Gland in the soles, massage the Heart in the left sole by using the manipulation changing from light to heavy and then to light again to stablize the heart rate. Tract and shake all the toes, press bellies of the toes with the nail border and push from the leg to the toes.

Remarks

1. The above point or zone groups are to be treated twice a day. Constant application of this massage has a better therapeutic effect on tachycardia caused by vegetative nerve functional disturbance.

2. This treatment may serve as a supplementary treatment for tachycardia caused by drugs, infection, fever, anemia, shock, cardiac failure, hyperthyroid heart disease and the cervical spondylopa-

thy of sympathetic type. Comprehensive treatments should be given to the original diseases according to their different conditions.

Anemia

When hemoglobin, red blood cell and packed cell volume in the circulatory blood are less or lower than normal, it is called anemia. Anemia is a common symptom in the clinic, which is of various types such as hemorralgic anemia, anemia due to anerythropoiesis (synthesis disturbance of hemoglobin or disturbance of nucleic maturity), and hemolytic anemia (including both the congenital hemolytic anemia and the hemolytic anemia after birth).

Essentials of Diagnosis

1. History of illness: Patient with acute hemolytic anemia usually has a traumatic history and patient with chronic hemolytic anemia often has a history of peptic ulcer, hemorrhoids, hookworm, menorrhage, etc. Patient with congenital hemolytic anemia usually has a family history and presents symptoms of the disease in the young age, while patient developing the hemolytic anemia in adult age usually suffers from the acquired hemolytic anemia.

2. Signs: Patient with a lowered blood pressure and shock usually has an acute hemorrahgic anemia; while one with fever, jaundice and splenomegaly has acute hemolytic anemia; chronic anemia is often indicated when patient has pale of the skin and mucous membrane, shortness of breath, enlargement of the heart and edema.

Massage Treatment

1. Precription of foot points: Press and knead bilateral Zusanli, Taixi, Sanyinjiao and Taichong; press with the nail border and knead bilateral Yinbai and Gongsun; and point and knead bilateral Yongquan.

2. Prescription of the foot reflecting zones: Press and knead the bilateral Stomach, Duodenum, Large Intestine and Thyroid Gland; press and point Kidney, Ureter, Bladder and Heart, Spleen and Liver in the left sole and the bilateral Cervical Vertebrae, Thoracic

Vertebrae, Lumbar Vertebrae and the Sacral Vertebra.

Remarks

1. The above prescribed groups of points or zones are to be treated twice a day. It is effective for the restoring stage of the hemorrhagic anemia and the anemia caused by peptic ulcer, dysfunctional uterine bleeding or malnutrition.

2. This therapy is not effective for pernicious anemia caused by aplastic anemia or malignant tumors.

Myocarditis

This is usually a flammatory manifestation of various kinds of systemic diseases in the cardiac muscles.

Essentials of Diagnosis

1. Patients with the disease often has such inflammatory diseases as viral infection, bacterial infection or parasitosis, a history of active rheumatism, a history of contacting chemical poisonous substances or some physical factors, or a history of allergic reaction.

2. The main symptoms of the disease include palpitation, shortness of breath, chest fullness, chest pain and the manifestations of the primary diseases. In a few patients, there is fever, cough, edema, nausea, or cardiac failure, cardiac shock, Admas-Strokes syndrome or even sudden death in severe cases.

3. Patients often have enlargement of the heart and weakened and blunt apex beats. In some cases, there is diastolic gallop rhythm, murmuring sound heard in different vulvular zones, arrhythmia and accelerated heart rate which is not proportional to the body temperature.

Massage Treatment

1. Prescription of the foot points: Press and knead bilateral Zusanli, Fenglong, Sanyinjiao, Taichong and Taixi; point and knead bilateral Jinggu; and knead and rub bilateral Yongquan.

2. Prescription of the foot reflecting zones: Press and knead Heart in the sole; point and press bilateral Adrenal Glands; push

and press Trachea in the soles and the Chest and Diaphragm on the dorsum of feet; and twist the 2nd and the 3rd toes of the feet.

Remarks

1. The above groups of points or zones are to be treated twice a day, which can relieve the symptoms of myocarditis.

2. This treatment is a supplementary therapy for myocarditis.

Rheumatic Heart Disease

This is also known as chronic rheumatic cardiac vulvopathy, which is caused by the lesion of the cardiac vulves following rheumatic carditis such as thickening and adhension of the vulves, adhesion of tendinous cords and papillary muscle or shortening of the tendinous cords to develop stenosis or insufficiency of the vulves. The mitral vulve, the aortic vulve and the tricuspid valve are the first three mostly frequently affected.

Essentials of Diagnosis

1. Clinical features

(1) Seen mostly in females aged from 15 to 40 years old.

(2) Patients with stenosis of the mitral vulve have palpitation, shortness of breath, coughing blood, or even dyspnea and orthpnea. In the advanced stage when right heart failure occurs, there are cyanotic lips and purplish cheeks, and diastolic murmur can be heard in the apex zone.

Patients with insufficiency of mitral vulve have lassitude, palpitation and dyspnea. When right heart failure occurs in the advanced stage, there is heaving apex impulse, and holosystolic murmur can be heard in the apex zone.

Patients with insufficiency of the aortic vulve have palpitation, shortness of breath, discomfort in the precardiac region and a throbbing feeling in head. When left heart failure occurs in the later stage, there is downward shifting of the apical impulse, heaving apex impulse, and holodiastolic murmur can be heard in the aortic region and the region of the 3rd and 4th ribs in the left border of sternum.

Patients with stenosis of the aortic vulve have lassitude, dizziness, dyspnea or even vertigo, syncope, angina pectoris or sudden death. When left heart failure occurs in the later stage, the apical impulse will shift downwards and to the left, and ejection murmur can be heard in the aortic zone.

Patients with combined valvular lesion have low fever, arthralgia, polyhidrosis, tachycardia which is not proportional to elevation of body temperature, and various kinds of complications.

Massage Treatment

1. Prescription of foot points: Press and knead the bilateral Zusanli, Yanglingquan, Fenglong, Taichong and Jinggu; rub and twist the 2nd and 3rd toes of the both feet; pinch and knead Zhongchong of the feet, and rub and knead Yongquan of the feet.

2. Prescription of the foot reflecting zones: Press and knead Heart in the sore of the left foot; push and press Adrenal Gland, Kidney, Ureter and Bladder in the soles of the two feet; point and knead Gallbladder in the sole of the right foot; and point and press the Chest and Diaphragm in the left foot.

Remarks

1. The above points are to be massaged twice a day. Constant application of this therapy can relieve symptoms of the rheumatic heart diseases.

2. This therapy can be adopted in combination with other therapies for severe rheumatic heart disease.

Pulmonary Heart Disease

This disease arises from chronic bronchial diseases, pulmonary diseases or thoracic diseases which causes increase of pulmonary circulation, hypertrophy of the right ventricle and the ensuing respiratory failure and heart failure.

Essentials of Diagnosis

1. This disease usually onsets in a cold weather.

2. Patients usually have a history of long-standing chronic cough with sputum or asthma. Lassitude and dyspnea usually occur in the later stage because the respiratory and circulatory functions can still be compensated in the early stage.

3. With progress of the disease, such symptoms as palpitation, aggravation of shortness of breath, or cyanosis will appear gradually, and heart failure and respiratory failure will develop eventually in the later stage. Besides, there is dysfunction of the nervous system, manifested as headache, restlessness, convulsion, tremor or even somnolence or coma.

Massage Treatment

1. Prescription of the foot point: Press and knead bilateral Zusanli, Fenglong and Neiting; point and knead bilateral Taixi and Duyin; pinch and knead bilateral Jinggu and Zhongchong; and knead and rub Yongquan.

2. Prescription of foot reflection zones: Pinch and press the Heart and the related Lymph zone in the left foot; constantly push and press the Adrenal Gland, Kidney, Ureter and Bladder of the two feet; and press and push the bilateral Lung and Trachea in the soles outwards.

Remarks

1. Massage the above points twice daily, and constant application of this therapy has a good effect for chronic bronchitis.

2. For cases with severe symptoms of heart failure, this therapy can be adopted as a supplementary treatment, and specific treatment must be given at the same time.

Sequela of Apoplexy

This condition, also called hemiplegia, is marked by paralysis in one side of the body.

Essentials of Diagnosis

1. Mostly caused by cerebral diseases. Such diseases as cerebral hemorrhage, cerebral embolism, cerebral thrombosis, traumatic in-

jury to brain and cerebral tumours often present deviation of mouth and eyes and hemiplegia after the acute stage.

2. Mainly manifested as motor dysfunction or diminution of decline of the sensory function in one side of the body, accompanied with deviation, aphasia, salivation, difficulty in swallowing and numbness of hands and feet.

Massage Treatment

1. Prescription of foot point: Press and knead Weizhong, Zusanli, Chengshan, Feiyang and Juegu in the affected side; press heavily Yinlingquan, Sanyinjiao, Qiuxu, Shangqiu, Taichong and Shenmai in the affected side; pinch and knead bilateral Zhongchong and Qiduan; and point and knead bilateral Yongquan.

2. Prescription of foot reflecting zones: Push and press Kidney, Ureter and Bladder in the soles of the two feet; point heavily the Heart in the left foot and the Liver in the right foot; and point and knead the bilateral Head.

Remarks

1. The above points are to be massaged once or twice a day with more strengthen exerted on the affected side.

2. This therapy should be applied as soon as possible after the acute stage of various kinds of cerebral accidents. It has a remarkable effect on helping patients recovery from hemiplegia, facial paralysis and aphasia.

Infection of the Upper Respiratory Tract

When the infection of virus or bacteria is limited in the nasal cavity or the pharynx and larynx, it is known as infection of the upper respiratory tract. This disease is usually mild, has a short course and a good prognosis, only a few patients may develop other diseases secondary to the infection.

Essentials of Diagnosis

1. This disease is mostly caused by virus, and bacterial infection is usually secondary to the viral infection. The induction factors in-

clude exposure to cold, being caught by rain and over fatigue.

2. Viral infection

(1) Common cold (affection of cold): Marked by acute rhinitis or catarrh symptoms of the upper respiratory tract, such as chills, general pantalgia, low fever, sneeze, stuffy nose and watery nasal discharge.

(2) Influenza: Severe in symptoms, clinically manifested as four types: the simple type, the pneumonia type, the toxic type and the gastrointestinal type.

(3) Viral infection with pharyngitis as the main manifestation.

In the case of viral infection, the WBC count is usually normal or a little lower than normal.

3. Bacterial infection: Being sudden in onset and manifested as chills, high fever, general aching, headache, sore throat and elevation of WBC count.

Massage Treatment

1. Prescription of foot points: Pinch and point bilateral Neiting, bilateral Shugu on the lateral sides of the feet, bilateral Zhaohai on the medial sides of the feet, Ludisanzhen on the soles of the feet and Sibai in the posterior side of the feet; press and knead the medial border of the dorsal side of the 2nd toe; and rub the soles.

2. Prescription of foot reflecting zones: Grasp the foot with the thumb and the index finger placed on depressions in the bilateral sides of the malleolus on the dorsal side of the foot, push and press upward the Lymph Gland of the Upper Body and the Lymph Gland of the Lower Body; point and knead the Thoracic Lymph Gland, Tonsil and the Lymph Gland of the Whole Body on the dorsal side of the feet; press and knead at the fixed reflecting zones of Frontal Sinus and Nose on the soles of the feet; push and press the Trachea; and point and knead the Spleen on the sole of the left foot.

Remarks

1. The above point or zone groups are to be massaged twice a day.

2. In a season with sudden climatic changes when common cold is likely to occur, application of this therapy once everyday has the ef-

fect of preventing cold.

Bronchitis

Bronchitis is divided into two types, the acute and the chronic. The former is usually caused by infection of virus or bacteria, or by physical or chemical substances which stimulate the mucous membrane of the bronchus.

Essentials of Diagnosis

1. Acute bronchitis: Being sudden in onset, manifested as chills, headache, moderate fever, general aching, rhinitis, hoarseness, irritative cough initially followed by expectoration of thin sputum which will become purulent and thick finally. If it attacks repeatedly, it will turn into a chronic one.

2. Chronic bronchitis: Most patients have a history of suffering from common cold, acute bronchitis, pneumonia, long-standing smoking or inhalation of irritative gases before developing the disease. Clinically it is manifested mainly by long-standing cough with sputum. The cough is usually severe in the morning and at night, mostly accompanied with viscious or foamy sputum. In severe cough, the sputum may be stained with blood occasionally. If infection follows, the sputum will increase in amount and become purulent in nature. Emphysema often results in chronic cases.

Massage Treatment

1. Prescription of foot points: Point and press bilateral Zusanli, Fenglong and Neiting; pinch and knead bilateral Taixi and Zhaohai; and pinch and press bilateral Lidui.

2. Prescription of foot reflecting zones: Point and press Accessory Thyroid Gland on the bilateral soles of feet; push transversely from the centers of Lung and Trachea toward their bilateral sides; point and press the Adrenal Gland on the bilateral soles; press and knead Throat, Trachea, Thoracic Lymph Gland, Lymph Gland of the Upper Body and Lymph Gland of the Lower Body on the dorsum of the feet.

Remarks

1. The above point or zone groups are to be treated twice a day. This therapy has a supplementary effect on the acute bronchitis, and it has a remarkable effect on helping patients with the chronic one recover from the disease if it is applied constantly.

2. Patients should prevent themselves from suffering from cold, avoid smoking and intake of alcohol, and do exercise to fortify the therapeutic effects.

Bronchial Asthma

This is a commonly seen and paroxysmal allergic disease of the respiratory tract. When it attacks, it will produce such symptoms as chest stuffiness, shortness of breath, asthma and cough as a result of spasm of the bronchial smooth muscles, the edema of mucous membrane complicated and the hypersecretion of the glands.

Essentials of Diagnosis

1. Patients have an allergic constitution and develop the disease due to contacting some sensibilisinogens such as inhalation or intake of some sensibilisinogens or infection of the respiratory tract.

2. In most cases, the disease has a sudden onset, with dyspnea, asthma, inability to lie flat and dry cough without sputum as the manifestations.

3. Rales can be heard in the lungs when the disease attacks. In chronic cases, the chest may become prominent and take a shape of barrel. If the disease repeatedly attacks, emphysema and pulmonary heart disease may result finally.

Massage Treatment

1. Prescription of foot points: Press and knead bilateral Zusanli and Fenglong; point and knead bilateral Taixi and Dazhong; knead heavily bilateral Yongquan; and rub the soles until they produce a hot feeling.

2. Prescription of the foot reflecting zones: Point and knead Accessory Thyroid Gland on the soles; push transversely Trachea and Lung on the soles; push continuously Kidney, Ureter and Bladder on the soles; push and press the Lymph Gland of the Upper Body on

the dorsum of the feet; and point and press the Thoracic Lymph Gland of the soles.

Remarks

1. The above point or zone groups are to be treated twice a day. The manipulation should be gradually aggravated from gentle to heavy at the onset stage of asthma, which has a remarkable asthma-relieving effect. Continuous application of this therapy can regulate flow of Qi, tonify the Lung, support Vital Qi and eliminate pathogens.

2. Patients should avoid intake of alcohol, fishy, acrid or pungent food, or the food that is likely to induce the disease. Besides, they should do proper out-door exercises.

3. When cardiac or pulmonary failure develops at the later stage of the disease, comprehensive therapeutic measures should be taken.

Stomachache

Stomachache may be seen in many diseases. The commonly encountered are the acute or chronic gastritis, peptic ulcer, and gastric neurosism. Its etiological factors include bacteria or bacterial toxin, stimuli of chemical substances or physical factors, improper diet, excessive eating or drinking, long-standing intake of irritative food, emotional stress, hypersecretion of gastric acid, etc, which cause the disease by stimulating the gastric mucous membrane and inducing spasm of the smooth muscles and disturbance of the gastrointestinal tract.

Essentials of Diagnosis

1. Acute gastritis: This condition has a sudden onset and is marked by discomfort, fullness, burning sensation or pain in the upper abdomen.

2. Chronic gastritis: This condition has a slow onset and is manifested as persistent pain in the upper abdomen. The pain is usually dull or is accompanied with a distension feeling in nature.

3. Peptic ulcer: The gastric ulcer is mostly seen in the small cur-

vature of the stomach, while the duodenal ulcer most affects the duodenal bulb. Clinically it is mainly marked by epigastric pain which is mostly dull pain, distending pain or burning pain in nature. The pain is rhythmic and attacks periodically, mostly in autumn and winter. Pain due to gastric ulcer mostly occurs $1\sim 2$ hours after eating, while pain due to duodenal ulcer is usually seen $2\sim 4$ hours after eating and will last until eating again. Pain in duodenal ulcer may also attack at night and can be relieved by eating in most cases, and it may radiate to the shoulder.

4. Gastrointestinal neurosism: In mild cases it is marked by discomfort with a burning sensation in the upper abdomen after eating, while in the severe cases, it may present severe stomachache, but it is not rhythmic and is often aggravated by anxiety, fright, terror or argument.

Massage Treatment

1. Prescription of foot points: Press, knead and point bilateral Liangqiu and Zusanli; point and knead bilateral Neiting, Gongsun and Taichong; rub Yongquan in the center of sole.

2. Prescription of foot reflecting zone: Press and knead bilateral Stomach and Duodenum; then press and push Kidney, Ureter, Bladder and Celiax Plexus.

Remarks

1. When the above point or zone groups are massaged with slightly heavy manipulations at the onset stage of the stomachache, they can relieve the pain markedly.

2. In the remission stage, the massage should be carried out according to the identified syndromes based on the prescription for the primary disease.

Vomiting

This is a reaction marked by adverse flow of the gastric content out of the mouth. Vomiting has two types, the central type and the peripheral type. The former is mainly seen in diseases with elevation of the intracranial pressure such as encephalitis, meningitis, hypertensive cerebral diseases and cerebral hemorrhage, diseases marked by vestibular functional disturbance such as vertigo syndrome or auditory vertigo, and diseases caused by emotional disturbance such as gastrointestinal neurosism or conditional reflex vomiting. It may also be induced by drugs or metabolic disturbance as seen in uremia and hypokalemia. The peripheral type is mostly seen in gastrogenic diseases such as acute or chronic gastritis, bacterial food poisoning, various types of gastritis or pyloric obstruction, or in such diseases as peritonitis, appendicitis, cholecystitis, pancreatitis and biliary ascariasis as a reflex activity of the stomach to the disease.

Essentials of Diagnosis

1. Age and occurrence of the disease: Vomiting in the aged is often a sign of gastric cancer; while that in the young or middle aged often indicates inflammation or obstruction of the digestive tract. The vomiting related to emotional changes is seen mostly in female. The acute vomiting often arises from inflammation or spasm of the digestive tract. And, slow vomiting with large amount of vomitus is mainly seen in pyloric obstruction.

2. Accompanying symptoms: Vomiting with fever is often seen in the early stage of some infectious diseases, that accompanied with severe headache mostly suggests elevation of the intracranial pressure, and that associated with colicky pain of the intestine may be seen in many different diseases of the digestive tract.

3. Vomiting with vibration of eyeballs, pale and lowering of blood pressure is usually seen in auditory vertigo; that accompanied with elevation of the intracranial pressure and the irritative symptoms of meninges is mainly seen in meningitis, brain tumor or cerebral hemorrhage; that of gastric pattern accompanied with a water-vibrating sound is usually seen in pyloric obstruction of various types; that of intestinal pattern with borborygmus is usually detected in intestinal obstruction of varying causes; and that with masses in the upper abdomen may be seen in hepatic cancer or gastric cancer.

Massage Treatment

1. Prescription of foot points: Press and knead bilateral Zusanli,

Taibai, Gongsun and Dadu; and point and knead Taichong and Yongquan.

2. Prescription of foot reflecting zones: Press and knead Stomach and Duodenum on the soles of feet; push and press bilateral Labyrinth and Head; rub transversely Diaphragm on the dorsal side of the feet; rub heavily the medial and lateral borders and the midline of the soles of feet.

Remarks

1. The above point or zone groups are to be treated twice a day. When vomiting attacks, this therapy has a better effect of relieving vomiting.

2. This therapy is extremely effective for vomiting caused by gastrointestinal neurosism. Vomiting caused by gastrointestinal tract should be treated with this therapy based on the syndromes identified, and constant application of this therapy has a better effect for the primary disease.

3. Vomiting caused by cerebral diseases or gastric cancer should be treated by taking other corresponding measures.

Phrenospasm

This is a disease marked by involuntary intermittent contraction of the diaphragm, which is mostly caused by inhalation of air into the respiratory tract with sudden close of the vocal fold. Besides, it may also be caused by gastric dilation, gastric neurosism and cerebral accidents due to stimuli of the vagus nerve or the ending of the phragmatic nerve, or by disorders of the central nervous system or emotional disturbance.

Essentials of Diagnosis

1. Hiccup which is frequent, short and rapid, lasting from several minutes to several hours. It may attack day and night or intermittently. In severe cases, it will influence speaking, chewing, breathing and sleeping, bringing about great suffering to patients.

2. When feeble hiccup occurs in patient with a long disease course

and a weak constitution associated with shortness of breath and cold limbs, it is often a sign of crisis.

Massage Treatment

1. Prescription of the foot points: Press and knead bilateral Zusanli, Taichong and Neiting; and pinch and point bilateral Zuqiaoyin.

2. Prescription of foot reflecting zones: Press and knead Stomach and Duodenum of the soles; point and press Thyroid Gland of the feet; press and knead the bilateral Celliac Plexus of soles; then press and knead Kidney, Ureter and Bladder; point and knead Throat and Trachea on the dorsum of feet; push and press the Diaphgram on the dorsum of feet; and rub the soles and dorsums of the feet until they produce a hotness sensation.

Remarks

1. The above point or zone groups are to be massaged twice daily. For hiccup caused by gastric neurosism, this treatment can relieve the hiccup at once.

2. This therapy can reduce frequency and severity of the hiccup that frequently occurs in the later and critical stage of some diseases, being valuable in alleviating patient's suffering when used together with other treatment measures.

Bacterial Dysentery

This is an acute intestinal infectious disease caused by dysentery bacillus, with pyogenic inflammation of the colon as its main pathological change.

Essentials of Diagnosis

1. Seen mostly in summer and autumn and having an acute onset.

2. Manifested as fever, abdominal pain and diarrhea which are accompanied with nausa, vomiting or even high fever, convulsion, coma and shock in severe cases.

3. Loose stool or watery stool with mucous fluid, followed by purulent and bloody stool and with notable tenesmus.

Massage Treatment

1. Prescription of foot points: Press and knead bilateral Zusanli, Yinlingquan and Shangjuxu; point and knead bilateral Neiting, Gongsun and Ludisanzhen; and pinch and knead Yongquan on the soles of feet.

2. Prescription of foot reflecting zones: Push and press Stomach and Duodenum of the soles; then push and press the Small Intestine of the soles; point and knead the Lymph Gland of the Upper Body and that of the Lower Body on the dorsum of feet; and then push and press Kidney, Ureter and Bladder. Push from the center of the heel toward the tips of the little toe and the big toe respectively along the lateral and the medial sides of the feet.

Remarks

1. The above point or zone groups are to be treated twice a day and are effective for acute bacterial dysentery.

2. Other therapies of both Chinese and Western medicine must be applied simultaneously for toxic dysentery with a sudden and critical condition.

Halitosis

This is a symtpom seen in many diseases.

Essentials of Diagnosis

1. A fetid smell from the mouth, which can be noted only by patient himself in mild cases and by others in severe cases.

2. Halitosis has many types. Halitosis with a sour and fetid smell often suggests diseases of the gastrointestinal tract; that with a fishy smell most indicates diseases of the respiratory tract; that with an apple smell usually signifies diabetes; that with a smell of decayed apple often indicates diseases of the respiratory tract; that with a urine smell indicates diseases of the kidney; that with a mouse smell mostly suggests liver diseases; and that with a bloody smell usually indicates bleeding of digestive tract, bronchiectasis, etc. In addition, dental caries may also result in halitosis.

Massage Treatment

1. Prescription of foot points: Press and knead bilateral Zusanli, Neiting, Lidui, Chongyang, Xingjian and Taichong, and Gongsun, Taibai and Taiyuan on the medial sides of the feet.

2. Prescription of foot massage zones: Push and press Stomach and Duodenum on the soles of the feet. Select different reflecting zones according to the different causative factors. That is, add Trachea and Lung for diseases of the respiratory tract; add Pancreas on the soles of the feet for diseases of the digestive tract; press and knead Liver on the left sole of the foot additionally for liver diseases; and add Kidney, Ureter and Bladder for diseases of the urinary system.

Remarks

1. The above point or zone groups are to be treated twice a day, and they may be applied in combination with the foot points or reflecting zones for primary diseases, which will bring about even better therapeutic effects.

2. Such corresponding measures as dental repairment must be taken for halitosis caused by dental caries.

Hyperhydrochloria

This is a disase marked by excessive secretion of gastric acid due to disturbance of the gastric secretion.

Essentials of Diagnosis

The typical manifestations of hyperhydrochloria include acid regurgitation, heartburning, fullness and distension in the epigastric region and the abdomen, acid eructation or eructation with a fetid odour, dry throat, bitter taste in the mouth, which are often accompnaied with spasmatic constipation, normal or excessive appetite, or stamachache that occurs 1~2 hours after eating.

Massage Treatment

1. Prescription of foot points: Press and knead bilateral Zusanli and Liangqiu; point and knead bilateral Neiting and Gongsun; and

pinch and knead bilateral Yinbai.

2. Prescription of foot reflecting zone: Push and press the Stomach and Duodenum of the soles; then push and press from Kidney to Bladder through Ureter; press with finger Celliac Plexus of the soles; and push transversely Diaphragm on the dorsums of feet; then, tract the big toe and rub the soles heavily.

Remarks

1. The above point or zone groups are to be treated twice a day. Better therapeutic effects can be obtained if the prescription for the primary diseases are adopted simultaneously.

2. Patient should keep his or her epigastric region warm, and avoid intake of such pungent, acrid or sweat foods as sweat potato, Chinese chives and the raw and cold food.

Chronic Gastritis

Here the chronic gastritis refers to the primary chronic gastritis which is caused by chronic stimuli and abnormality of the gastric wall. According to the pathologic changes of the gastric mucous membrane, it can be divided into the chronic superficial gastritis, the chronic atrophic gastritis and the chronic hypertrophic gastritis.

Essentials of Diagnosis

1. In most cases, the following etiological factors often exist before occurrence of the disease:

(1) Chronic stimuli: Intake of hard and thick food, excessive smoking, intake of strong alcohol, strong tea or coffee, intake of too hard or hot, pungent or acrid food and dysfunction of the pylorus.

(2) Disturbance of the gastric wall: Damage of the gastric mucous membrane, congestion of the gastric mucous membrane, insufficiency of gastric acid, disturbance of the endocrine system and poor auto-immunity.

2. It has a slow onset and a slow development with a long illness course and without special symptoms.

3. The superficial gastritis is mainly manifested as discomfort, fullness or pain in the upper abdomen accompanied with eructation.

4. The atrophic gastritis usually exhibits poor appetite, discomfort in the upper abdomen, diarrhea, emaciation, anemia, glossitis or atrophy of the tongue.

5. The hypertrophic gastritis is mainly marked by pain in the upper abdomen, which is not periodic nor regular, mostly accompanied with acid regurgitation, eructation and tenderness in the upper abdomen.

6. This disease may be complicated by peptic ulcer, gastrodialysis, gastric cancer, bleeding of the upper digestive tract, etc.

Massage Treatment

1. Prescription of foot points: Press and knead bilateral Zusanli, Neiting, Taichong and Gongsun; and point and knead bilateral Yongquan.

2. Prescription of foot reflecting zones: Push and preass Stomach and Duodenum on the soles of feet; press Thyroid Gland and Celliac Plexus at fixed spots on the soles of feet; press Spleen on the left sole with finger; push and press from Kidney to Bladder through Ureter on the soles of the feet; and push and press the Upper and the Lower Lymph Gland on the dorsums of the feet. In addition, rub the soles heavily and stamp the soles.

Remarks

1. The above point or zone groups are to be treated twice a day. If self-massage is carried out by kneading the upper abdomen 30~50 cycles clockwise and counterclockwise respectively, the therapeutic effects will be even better.

2. Food raw, cold, pungent and acrid, difficult to be digested as well as alcohol and smoking are forbidden.

Gastric and Duodenal Ulcer

This is a diseases caused by comprehensive causes, which is related to inheridity, stimuli of chemical or physical factors and some diseases. Under the action of these factors, the erosion effect of the gastric acid and the gastric pepsin is strengthened and the defensive function of the gastric mucosa is weakened, so ulcer results.

Essentials of Diagnosis

1. Seen mostly in young and middle aged people and in autumn and winter, and slow in onset.

2. Mainly manifested as pain in the upper abdomen which may be complicated by eructation, acid regurgitation, nausea, vomiting, constipation, etc.

3. The pain in the upper abdomen has a slow and periodic onset, regurlarly related to eating and is usually relieved by eating or administration of alkaline drugs.

4. Pain of gastric ulcer occurs in the middle or a little left below the xiphoid process and $1\sim2$ hours after eating, and usually disappears before next meal; while that of duodenal ulcer often presents in the middle or a little right below the xiphoid process which occurs $2\sim4$ hours after eating. Usually it is relieved when next meal is completed and it has notable acid regurgitation.

5. Patients with so severe pain that influences eating may be complicated by loss of weight, mild tenderness in the upper abdomen, or even bleeding, perforation, pyloric obstruction or canceration.

Massage Treatment

1. Prescription of foot points: Press and knead bilateral Zusanli, Liangmen and Yinlingquan; point and knead Neiting, Gongsun, Taichong, and Ludisanzhen on the soles; and press and rub bilateral Yongquan.

2. Prescription of foot reflecting zone: Push and press the Stomach and the Duodenum on the soles of feet; push and press from Kidney to Bladder through Ureter; point and knead Pituitary Gland on the soles of feet; press and knead Liver on the right sole; and press and knead Celliac Plexus on the soles of feet. Besides, rub heavily the medial and lateral borders and the soles of feet.

Remarks

1. The above point or zone groups are to be treated twice a day. Constant application of this therapy has a better effect on rehabilita-

tion of ulcer patients.

2. Patients should live a regular life, combine rest with work organically, regulate his or her diet, keep an open mind and avoid overfatigue.

Chronic Diarrhea

This is a common symptom in the clinic, which refers to increase of defecation frequency with loose stools or a stool with pus and blood or mucous fluid. There are many factors causing diarrhea. Diseases of the stomach, intestine, pancreas and gallbladder can all give rise to the disease, but it is mostly seen in inflammation of the intestine. Emotional stress, excitement, disturbance of endocrine system, intestinal indigestion, disturbance of blood circulation in intestine, allergic reaction of the intestine or poisoning of chemical drugs can also cause the disease.

Essentials of Diagnosis
1. Diarrhea is divided into two types: the acute and the chronic. The acute refers to the diarrhea with a sudden onset and an illness course shorter than 2 months; while the chronic indicates the diarrhea with a slow onset, repeated attacks and an illness course longer than 2 months.

2. The acute diarrhea is marked by several or even more than 10 times of defecation a day with a loose or sour and fetid stool, poor appetite, borborygmus, abdominal pain, vexation, thirst, scanty and dark urine with a hot sensation, burning sensation in anus. If the stool contains pus and blood and is complicated with tenesmus, it indicates bacterial infection.

3. Chronic diarrhea: Several defecations a day, alternate occurrence of onset and remission of the condition, poor appetite, lassitude, sallow complexion, loss of weight, or even edema of face and limbs. Diarrhea is often aggravated by eating greasy food.

Massage Treatment
1. Prescription of foot points: Press and knead bilateral Zusanli,

Shangjuxu and Chengshan; point and knead bilateral Neiting, Taichong, Jiexi and Gongsun; and push and rub the midline of the soles.

2. Prescription of foot reflecting zones: Push and press Stomach and Duodenum on the soles, push and press Large Intestine along the direction of colon; press with finger the Small Intestine and Celliac Plexus on the soles; and push and press the Upper and Lower Lymph Gland on the dorsum of feet.

Remarks

1. The above point or zone groups are to be treated twice a day, which has a better effect on the chronic diarrhea caused by commonly seen digestive diseases and the diarrhea caused by gastrointestinal neurosism.

2. Better therapeutic effect can be obtained if the abdomen is rubbed counterclockwise with umbilicus as the center, 50 times each time, twice a day, in combination with the above therapy.

Constipation

Constipation is a morbid condition marked by dry stool, prolonged retention of stool in the intestine, reduce of the defecation frequency or absence of defecation in 2 days. This disease may be caused by many factors. If it is caused by weakened peristalsis of the colon and the ensuing slow movement of the food residue in the colon, it is a colon constipation; and if it is caused by prolonged retention of food residue in the rectum, it is a constipation of rectum. Constipation also includes occasional constipation which arises from delayed treatment of the occasional constipation and most rectal constipation falls into this category. Habitual constipation usually arises from inadequacy of the power to discharge faeces due to general weakness, chronic disease, insufficient exercise or ageing and most colon constipation belongs to this category.

Essentials of Diagnosis

1. Dry and hard stool with difficult discharge of faece, abdominal

fullness, eructation, poor appetite, headache, dizziness, insomnia, chest fullness, irritability, sallow complexion, dry lips, and scanty and dark urine. Long-standing constipation may result in hemorrhoids or anal fissure.

2. Alternate occurrence of constipation and diarrhea is often seen in intestinal tuberculosis, or colon allergy. If constipation is also complicated by bright red blood in the stools and emaciation, it often indicates colon cancer or rectal cancer. If this condition is accompanied with abdominal pain, vomiting or abdominal masses, it usually signifies intestinal obstruction.

Massage Treatment

1. Prescription of foot points: Press and knead bilateral Zusanli, Shangjuxu and Xingjian; point and knead Taixi, Zhaohai and Dazhong; and pinch and knead bilateral Ludisanzhen and Yongquan.

2. Prescription of foot reflecting zones: Push and press Stomach, Duodenum and Pancreas on bilateral soles; push and press Large Intestine and Accessory Thyroid Gland on the soles along the direction of the colon; and knead and twist Rectum and Anus above the medial malleolus of the feet.

Remarks

1. The above point or zone groups are to be treated twice a day. If it is conducted together with massaging the abdomen clockwise with the umbilicus as the centre, which is to be performed 50 times each time, 1~2 times daily, it will have a better effect.

2. Patient shoud take a cup of diluted saline water in the early morning, eat more vegetable or fruit, avoid intake of pungent, acrid or irritative food, and defecate at a regular time.

3. This therapy is ineffective for constipation due to intestinal tuberculosis or cancer.

Gastroptosis

This indicates downward shifting of the location of the stomach, which is mostly caused by lowering of the abdominal pressure due to

relaxation of abdominal wall.
Essentials of Diagnosis
1. Mostly seen in patients with weak constitution or malnutrition and women with multiple deliveries. Its main symptoms include abdominal fullness which is aggravated by eating and relieved by lying flat, accompanied with abdominal distending pain, loose or dry stool, poor appetite, lassitude, palpitation, dizziness or faint.

2. The lower abdomen droops and is enlarged when taking a standing position, while it will disappear in a lying position. Strong abdominal aortic throbbing can be felt in the upper abdomen, and ptosis of liver or kidney may be complicated sometimes.

Massage Treatment
1. Prescription of foot points: Press and knead bilateral Zusanli, Neiting, Taichong and Chongyang, and pinch and knead bilateral Yinbai and Shangqiu.

2. Prescription of foot reflecting zone: Press and knead Stomach and Duodenum on the soles of the feet; push transversely Diaphragm on the dorsum of the feet laterally, rub the center of soles and push and press along the midpoint of the heel to the midline of the soles.

Remarks
1. The above point or zone groups are to be treated twice a day. Constant application of this therapy has a better effect.

2. Patient should live a regular life, keep a pleasant mood, and avoid intake of excessive raw, cold or irritative food or the food that is difficult to digest.

3. As supplementary measures, patient should do such exercise as sit-ups to exercise the abdominal muscles.

Gastrointestinal Neurosism

This is a functional disturbance of the stomach and intestine caused by functional dysturbance of the high nervous system with disordered secretion and movement of the stomach and intestine as the main pathologic changes. It is usually inorganic but it may occur as a sequela of organic diseases of the gastrointestinal tract.

Essentials of Diagnosis

1. In most cases, it has a slow onset, being persistent or intermittent, with a generally good conditions.

2. Gastric neurosism is usually manifested as anorexia, eructation, acid regurgitation, hiccup, nausea, vomiting, and burning sensation, fullness or pain in the upper abdomen.

3. Intestinal neurosism: It is mainly marked by the symptoms commonly seen in diseases of the intestinal tract such as abdominal pain or discomfort, abdominal fullness, borborygmus, diarrhea and constipation. The allergic colon is usually marked by motor disturbance in most cases, manifested as paroxysmal colicky pain in the left lower abdomen, abdominal fullness, constipation and frequent wind breaks. Intestinal neurosism with secretion disturbance is rare and it is mainly manifested as diarrhea, loose stools with much mucous fluid and tenesmus. Secretion and motor disturbances may occur together or alternately.

4. Apart from mild migratory tenderness in the upper abdomen, hepatic or splenic flexures of colon and left lower abdomen and spasmic intestinal tract in the lower abdomen, no other positive sign can be revealed.

5. It is accompanied with such symptoms of neurosism as insomnia, forgetfulness, dream-disturbed sleep, anxiety, lassitude, palpitation, chest stuffiness and hypersensitivity of the nerve.

Massage Treatment

1. Prescription of foot points: Press and knead bilateral Zusanli, Neiting and Taichong; point and knead bilateral Zhaohai and Gongsun; pinch and knead bilateral Lidui and Yinbai; and press and knead Shangjuxu, Xiajuxu and Sanyinjiao additionally for intestinal neurosism.

2. Prescription of foot reflecting zones: Pinch and knead Frontal Sinus, Cerebrum and Cerebellum of the feet toe by toe; push and press from Kidney to Bladder through Ureter on the feet; press and knead Celliac Plexus, Stomach, Duodenum and the Lower Ab-

domen.
Remarks
1. The above point or zone groups are to be treated twice a day and have a better therapeutic effects for the disease.
2. Although this disease has some typical clinical manifestations, organic diseases must be excluded when making the diagnosis.

Viral Hepatitits

This is an infectious disease of the digestive tract caused by hepatitis viruses which are usually classified as four types, A, B, C and D. Diffusive swelling, degeneration, necrosis and regeneration of the hepatic cells are the main pathologic changes of the disease.

Essentials of Diagnosis
1. Hepatitis A: It is caused by virus of hepatitis A, affected through the mouth, has a short petential period and an acute attack. Most patients experience a sudden onset which is marked by fever, yellow slcera and skin, dark brown urine, nausea after eating fatty food, pain in the hepatic region, lassitude, remarkable elevation of GPT and a positive result in urobilin and cholirubin examination.
2. Hepatitis B: This is a disease caused by virus of hepatitis B which affects human body by means of blood transfusion, injection of serum products and the sinringe and unstrictly disinfected needles in acupuncture, or by the mother-fetus means or direct comtamination. It has a long incubation period, a slow onset and patients often have lassitude, poor appetite, dulling pain in the liver region and abnormal liver function. Most patients have not jaundice. This disease has a long illness course and tends to attack repeatedly or become chronic active hepatitis or chronic persistent hepatitis. In some cases, it may develop into cirrhosis of liver or liver cancer.

Massage Treatment
1. Prescription of foot points: Press and knead bilateral Zusanli and Sanyinjiao; press and knead bilateral Taichong and Zhongfeng at fixed points; pinch and twist the medial and lateral borders of the

big toes; and rub bilateral Yongquan.

2. Prescription of foot reflecting zones: Press and knead Liver and Gallbladder on the soles of feet and the Spleen on the left foot; press and push from Kidney to Bladder through Ureter; push and press Upper Lymph Gland and Lower Lymph Gland on the dorsum of feet; point and press Liver Meridan Gland; and push and press Thoracic Lymph Gland.

Remarks

1. The above point or zone groups are to be treated twice a day. It is helpful in rehabilitation of the chronic hepatitis.

2. This therapy may be adopted as a supplementary therapy for the acute hepatitis or cirrhosis of liver and liver cancer developed from the advanced hepatitis.

Cholecystitis and Cholelithiasis

These two diseases are commonly seen acute abdomen. Cholecystitis is an inflammatory disease of the gallbladder caused by bacterial infection and stimuli of the concentrated bile or the pancreatic fluid that flows back into the gallbladder and it is usually divided into the acute type and the chronic type. Cholelithiasis is a disease marked by symptoms caused by stone in the gallbladder or the biliary tract, which is mostly related to the core of stone caused by infection of the gallbladder, retention of bile, disturbance of cholesterol and the fragments of the roundworm.

Essentials of Diagnosis

1. Acute cholecystitis: Persistent pain in the right hypochondrium and upper abdomen, which is aggravated gradually and radiates to the right shoulder and scapular region, accompanied with nausea, vomiting, increased muscular tension in the affected zone and palpable gallbladder sometimes. When angiocholitis is complicated, there will be jaundice, yellow sclera, yellow and scanty urine, and constipation. If the bile duct is obstructed completely, grey white stools will be detected.

2. Chronic cholecystitis: This condition may be transformed from the acute cholecystitis, or caused by chronic stimuli of the stone in the gallbladder. It is usually marked by indigestion, gastric fullness, eructation, acid regurgitation, discomfort in the upper or right upper abdomen, persistent dull pain or pain in the right scapular region. These symptoms are usually intractable, although they may not be so severe, and a mild dull pain in the gallbladder is often experienced.

3. Cholelithiasis: Paroxysmal colicky pain in the upper abdomen or the right rib border, which may sometimes radiate to the back or the right shoulder, nausea, reflex vomiting, increased abdominal muscular tension, jaundice in most cases, grey white stools, and strong tea-like urine. When pericholecystitis, peritonitis or empyema of gallbladder is complicated, there will be chills and high fever; and if the obstruction lasts a long time, it may develop cirrhosis of the liver.

Massage Treatment

1. Prescription of foot points: Press and knead bilateral Yanglingquan and Dannangxue; point and knead bilateral Taichong and Gongsun; and pinch and knead bilateral Xiaxi and Zuqiaoyin.

2. Prescription of the foot reflecting zones: Push and press Liver and Gallbladder on the left sole and the Stomach and Duodenum on the bilateral soles; press and push the Lymph Gland of the Upper Body, the Lymph Gland of the Lower Body and the Thoracic Lymph Gland.

Remarks

1. The above point or zone groups are to be treated twice a day. This therapy has a good pain-relieving effect for acute cholecystitis and should be adopted in combination with other therapies according to changes of the illness conditions and the complications. Surgical treatments should be given in time. When the gallbladder and the biliary duct presents presymptoms of diabrosis, necrosis or perforation, ascaridol should be given in ascariasis of the biliary duct after pain is relieved.

2. Patients should have a regular diet and avoid sudden excessive

eating or drinking and excessive intake of the food containing much fat or cholesterol.

Edema

This is a disease marked by abnormal fluid retention in the tissue spaces out of the vessels caused by many factors, which is divided into the general edema and the localized edema. The general edema may be seen in cardiopathy, kidney diseases, liver diseases, malnutrition, diseases of the connective tissues and diseases of the endocrine system; while the localized edema is mainly seen in local inflammation, disturbed venous return, disturbed lymphatic return and angioneural edema.

Essentials of Diagnosis

1. General edema: If it starts in the lower position of the body and is accompanied with signs or symptoms of the cardiac diseases, it is a cardiac edema; if it occurs in the eyelids or face and is accompanied with symptoms of the kidney diseases, it is a renal edema; if it presents ascites first and then edema of the limbs with the manifestations of the liver diseases, it is a hepatic edema; general edema with manifestations of malnutrition or anemia indicates a malnutritive edema. Diseases of the connective system and the endocrine system may also exhibit general edema. A long-standing general edema without a known cause is usually idiopathic edema. If patients have notable obesity after the edema is relieved, the edema may be an obesity edema; and the gravity edema is mainly seen in people standing working long or travelling long.

2. Localized edema: If redness and obvious tenderness are found in a local zone with edema, it is a local edema due to allergic reaction or inflammation. If it is seen in the leg of one side, it may indicate venous engorgement, thrombophebitis and thrombosis. If the edema is seen in the face and upper part of the chest and is accompanied with dilation of the cervical vein and the chest wall, it may indicate superior vena cava syndrome. If the edema looks like elephant skin, it indicates filariasis.

Massage Treatment

1. Prescription of foot points: Press and knead bilateral Zusanli, Yinlingquan and Weiyang; point and knead bilateral Fuliu, Taixi, Taichong and Zhaohai; and pinch and knead bilateral Dadu, Gongsun and Ludisanzhen.

2. Prescription of foot reflecting zones: Point Adrenal Gland of the feet, Liver on the right sole and Heart and Spleen on the left sole; push and knead from Kidney to Bladder through Ureter; push and press Lymph Gland of the Upper Body and Lymph Gland of the Lower Body on the dorsum of the feet; and point and knead Thoracic Lymph Gland. Besides, rub the midline of foot, centers of the feet and heels heavily.

Remarks

1. The above point or zone groups are to be treated twice a day. This therapy is effective for edema of varying causes at their early stage, but it is not effective for severe edema seen in the later stage of the primary diseases.

2. When this therapy is to be adopted, the cause of the edema must be identified in time so that corresponding treatment can be given in time according to the primary diseases.

Infection of the Urinary System

This is a group of diseases caused by bacteria which enter the urinary system through blood stream, lymphatic fluid or the urinary tract, of which acute cystitis and acute or chronic pyelonephritis are most commonly seen. Secondary infection is likely to occur. For example, pyelonephritis may cause cystitis by means of descending infection; while cystitis can cause pyelonephritis by means of ascending infection. Obstruction, traumatic injury, stone or deformity of the urinary tract often induce onset of the disease. Invasion of bacteria into the urinary tract may cause symptoms of the urinary tract or cystitis and may go up further to affect the kidney. This disease is usually caused by haemetogenous spread, lymph tube spread or spread of the adjacent infections.

Essentials of Diagnosis

1. Acute or chronic pyelonephritis: The acute pyelonephritis is mainly marked by chills, high fever, headache, heaviness of the body, lassitude, poor appetite, occasional nausea, vomiting or the accompanying symptoms of infection of the upper respiratory tract, lumbago, pain in the abdomen or in the lower abdomen, frequent, urgent or painful urination, gross hematuria, percussion pain in the kidney region and tenderness in the urethra. If the acute fails to be cured for a long time, it may turn into the chronic which is manifested as such infectious symptoms of the urinary tract as mild but frequent urgent, frequent and painful urination with a burning sensation and low fever. The chronic pyelonephritis tends to attack repeatedly but it doesn't present acute attack.

2. Acute and chronic cystitis: The acute cystitis is mainly manifested as frequent, urgent and painful urination, pyuria or hematuria, without general symptoms in most cases. The chronic cystitis is more commonly seen than the acute one and it is mainly manifested as irritative symptoms of the bladder such as urgent, frequent and painful urination, spasmatic tenesmus sometimes, or terminal hematuria, turbid urine, and pyeuria in severe cases. In most cases, there is no general symptom.

Massage Treatment

1. Prescription of the foot points: Push and knead bilateral Yinlingquan and Sanyinjiao; point and knead bilateral Taixi, Fuliu and Taichong; pinch and knead bilateral Rangu and Yinbai; and knead and rub bilateral Yongquan.

2. Prescription of foot reflecting zones: Push and press from Kidney to Bladder through Ureter on the soles of the feet; push and knead Spleen on the sole of the left foot; push and press Lymph Gland of the Lower Body and Thoracic Lymph Gland on the dorsum of the feet; and push and press Ureter in the medial side of the heels of the feet.

Remarks

1. The above point or zone groups are to be treated twice a day.

This therapy has a better effect of clearing away heat, relieving inflammation and strengthening the urinary function of the kidney.

2. Women should keep their external genitalia clean and pay attentions to menstrual hygiene, and diapper for babies should be changed frequently in order to avoid urinary tract infection.

Chronic Glomerulonephritis

This disease, also briefly known as chronic nephritis, mostly arises from repeated attack of acute glomerulonephritis and is mainly seen in adults. It onsets slowly and progresses rapidly or slowly. At the advanced stage, it may develop chronic renal failure.

Essentials of Diagnosis
1. The typical manifestations of the disease include hematuria, proteinuria, cast urine, edema and hypertension. Other manifestations include a normal fundus or pale of retina and thinning of the arteries on the fundus, lassitude, unconcentration, aversion to cold or heat, etc.

2. In mild cases, there is small amount of proteinuria or microscopic hematuria, while in severe cases, there are anemia and severe hypertension or even development of renal failure.

Massage Treatment
1. Prescription of foot points: Press and knead bilateral Yinlingquan, Taixi and Sanyinjiao; point and knead bilateral Fuliu, Rangu and Gongsun; pinch and knead bilateral Ludisanzhen of feet; and rub and twist Yongquan of feet.

2. Prescription of foot reflecting zones: Push and press Adrenal Gland and from Kidney to Bladder through Ureter on the soles; point and knead Spleen on the left sole, push and press Lymph Gland of Upper Body and Lymph Gland of Lower Body on the dorsum of feet.

Remarks
1. The above point or zone groups are to be treated twice a day. Constant application of this therapy is helpful for rehabilitation of

patients with chronic glomerulonephritis.

2. Patients should have a good rest in a silent environment and avoid exposure to wind or cold, over fatigue or intake of salt or fatty and greasy food or the sea products.

3. Patients should give up smoking or intake of alcohol and have less sexual intercourses.

Enuresis

This means involuntary discharge of urine during sleep in children at the school age, which is caused by failure to cultivate a better sanitorial habit in the very young age of the children, or by organic diseases in a few cases. If a child is used to passing urine with a vague mind during sleeping as a result of long-standing urination in a vague mind due to laziness or drinking too much in the evening or being too tired, it is not a morbid condition. According to TCM, this disease is mainly caused by deficiency of the Kidney Qi and the ensuing failure of the Bladder to be controlled.

Essentials of Diagnosis

1. This disease mostly affects the children below 15 years old.

2. The main symptom is involuntary urine discharge during sleep, which mostly occurs at midnight or before dawn, once every night or even several times a night. Long-standing enuresis in adults is mostly caused by organic diseases.

Massage Treatment

1. Prescription of foot points: Press and knead Zusanli and Yinlingquan; point and knead bilateral Sanyinjiao, Taixi and Zhaohai; pinch and press bilateral Sibai on the posterior side of soles and Yejing of the feet; and rub Yongquan in the sole.

2. Prescription of foot reflecting zones: Push and press from Kidney to Bladder through Ureter; press and knead Cerebellum and Brain Steam; press and knead Heart on the sole of the left foot; press or knead Lymph Gland of Upper Body and Lymph Gland of Lower Body; push Uterus and Prostrate with the thumb extending

straight or flexed in the medial side of dorsum of feet. In addition, rub soles of feet powerfully, and push the zone behind the medial malleolus from the toes to the lower leg.

Remarks

1. The above point or zone groups are to be treated twice a day, which has a better effect for enuresis.

2. Organic diseases causing enuresis such as deformity of urinary tract should be treated positively.

3. Parents should cooperate well with doctors during treatment. They should give less water to their children in evening and wake up the children to pass urine at regular times so that the children can gradually get habit to get up to pass urine.

Retention of Urine

Filling of large volume of urine in bladder and failure of the urine to be discharged is known as retention of urine. Retention of urine caused by disorders of the central nerves or nervous injury, such as tumours of the spinal cord or the brain and myolesclerosis, is called nervous urine retention. If it is caused by pain of the ureter, prostrate gland or anus or hysteria, it is called reflex urine retention. And, if it is caused by stenosis or stone of the ureter or hypertrophy of prostrate gland, it is termed mechanical urine retention.

Essentials of Diagnosis

1. This disease is mainly seen in patients with the above-mentioned diseases, especially the aged patients with hypertrophy of the prostrate gland or the patients lying flat long after operation.

2. It often occurs suddenly, manifested as knuckle in the middle of the lower abdomen, excessive filling of the bladder, strong desire for urination but failure to urinate, persistent distending pain in the lower abdomen with great suffering, restlessness, moaning and fright.

3. When excessive filling of the bladder caused by acute or chronic urine retention brings about paralysis of the bladder wall, or

if the urine retention is caused by injury of the central nerve, patient may present no or only mild symptoms.
Massage Treatment
1. Prescription of foot points: Press and knead bilateral Yinlingquan and Sanyinjiao, point and knead bilateral Taixi, Taichong and Dazhong; and pinch and press Yongquan of the feet.
2. Prescription of foot reflecting zones. Press and knead from Kidney to Bladder through Ureter and Genital Gland; push with only one thumb the medial sides of the feet from the heels to Prostrate Gland and push Ureter upwards. In addition, rub the midline of the soles and tract and shake toes of the two feet.
Remarks
1. The above point or zone groups are to be treated twice a day. In addition, abdomen-rubbing may be done clockwise in the lower abdomen, 30~50 times each time. This therapy has a better therapeutic effect on reflex urine retention.
2. The primary diseases should be treated in patients with mechanical urine retention.

Hyperthyroidism

This is a disease caused by auto-immunoloy which produces the thyroid stimulation immunologic globulin and emotional injury which causes proliferation of the thyroid gland and the excessive secretion of thyroxin.
Essentials of Diagnosis
1. Seen mostly in female and in the population of 20~40 years old. It usually has a slow onset, and only a few of the patients may experience sudden onsets due to emotional injury or infection.
2. Manifestations of excessive secretion of thyroxin, including symptoms of increase of excitability of the sympathetic nerve and increase of the metabolism such as restlessness, being talkative, liability to be excited, fine and rapid tremor of fingers and tongue, weakness of muscles, persistent acceleration of heart beats, eleva-

tion of systolic pressure, lowering of the diastolic pressure, increase of difference between systolic and diastolic pressures, premature heart beats, paroxysmal tachycardia, atrial fibrillation, excessive appetite, frequent defecations, emaciation, aversion to hotness, warm and wet skin and profuse sweating.

3. The thyroid enlargement is usually mild or moderate diffusive enlargement accompanied with tremor and vascular murmur.

4. Exophthalmus is usually mild bilateral symmetric prominence of the eyeballs, with widened eye fissures, bright piercing eyes or staring eye. It may also be more prominent in one eye.

Massage Treatment

1. Prescription of the foot points: Press and knead Zusanli, Sanyinjiao; point and knead bilateral Kunlun and Zulinqi; and rub Yongquan with more force.

2. Prescription of foot reflecting zone: Press bilateral Pituitary Gland, Adrenal Gland, Kindey, Ureter and Bladder from upper part to lower part part at fixed points; push and press Thyroid Gland, Accessory Thyroid Gland and Genital Gland from lower part to upper part of the soles; and push and press Heart in the left sole and Lymph Gland of the Upper Body on the dorsum of feet.

Remarks

1. The above point or zone groups are to be treated twice a day. Constant application of this therapy has a better therapeutic effect on controlling the further development and relieving the symptoms of the disease.

2. Patient should eat more sea-tangle, fish, shrimp or mushroom and avoid emotional stimuli.

Diabetes

This is a commonly seen metabolic endocrine disease with a heriditary tendency, which is caused by relatively or absolutely inadequate secretion of insulin and excessive secretion of enteroglucogen and the ensuing disturbance of sugar metabolism. It may be related to auto-immunity, viral infection or heriditary factors.

Essentials of Diagnosis

1. Often induced by heriditary factor, obesity, excessive eating, inadequate exercise, emotional stimuli, frequent pregnancy, infection, operation, traumatic injury or application of adrenal cortex hormones.

2. It may onset at any age, but mostly seen in 40~60 years old and rarely seen below 15 years old.

3. It onsets slowly, and no obvious symptoms can be noted at the early stage or in mild cases. The typical symptoms are polyuria, excessive drinking and hyperphagia, lassitude, emaciation or loss of weight. The secondary symptoms include itching in external genitalia or the whole body, soreness and numbness of the limbs, pain in the back or lower back, irregular menstruation, etc.

Massage Treatment

1. Prescription of foot points: Press and push bilateral Zusanli and Sanyinjiao; point and knead bilateral Taichong, Neiting and Taixi; pinch and knead bilateral Shuiquan and Rangu; and rub heavily bilateral Yongquan.

2. Prescription of foot reflecting zone: Push and press from Stomach to Pancreas through Duodenum on the soles of feet; point and knead Adrenal Gland of the soles of feet; push and press from Kidney to Bladder through Ureter; push transversely Lung and Trachea on the soles; and push and press the Lymph Gland of the Upper Body and the Lymph Gland of the Lower Body on the dorsal side of feet from upper to lower.

Remarks

1. The above point or zone groups are to be treated twice a day, which has a better effect on diabetes.

2. The complicated complications of the disease should be treated by adopting the relevant prescriptions in concerning diseases.

3. Patient should control his or her diet, reduce his or her weight and avoid emotional stimuli.

Menopausal Syndrome

This refers to a group of syndromes marked by functional disturbance of the vegetative nerve in a period of time before or after natural menopause or due to loss of ovary function following surgical insection or radiotherapy. This disease may be mild, severe, long or short, and the critical case, which will influence one's life and work, should be given proper treatment in order to help patient go through this period smoothly.

Essentials of Diagnosis

1. Changes of menstruation: Disordered menstrual cycles, less mense, shortened menstrual period or menorrhagia. In some cases, it is manfiested as delayed menstruation, metrorrhagia and increased mense volume, followed by irregular or sudden stoppage of menstruation.

2. Functional disturbance of the psycho-nerve system: Mainly disturbance of the vegetative nerve which may present as: paroxysmal flushed face, distending pain in the head and neck, irritability which is more severe after eating, accompanied with sweating, aversion to cold, restlessness or poor sleep in severe case due to dysfunction of the vaso-nerve, especially hyperactivity of the cervical sympathetic nerve; irritability marked by liability to get nervous and excited, insomnia, lassitude and mental depression; skin numbness or itching with a sensation of ant creeping, headache, arthralgia or aching in the back and the low back; or dizziness, vertigo, tinnitus, vomiting, unconcentration of mind or decline of memory in a few cases.

3. Functional disturbance of the cardiovascular system: Palpitation, tachycardia or bradycardia, elevation or great variation of the blood pressure.

4. Metabolic disturbance: Fat metabolic disturbance manifested as obesity, especially in the loin, abdomen and hip; sugar metabolic disturbance marked by elevation of blood sugar, urine sugar detected with ocassional excessive appetite or easy to get hungery,

water and salt metabolic disturbance with frequent retentive edema of varying degrees; and disturbance of phosphrous and calcius metabolism marked by osteoporosis, decalcification of bone and liability to be fractured.

5. Changes of sexual organs: Atrophy of external genitalia with thinning of endomembrane and a tendency to develop vagititis.

Massage Treatment

1. Prescription of the foot points: Press and knead bilateral Zusanli and Sanyinjiao; point and knead bilateral Taixi, Taichong and Gongsun; pinch and knead bilateral Zhaohai and Yinbai; and rub bilateral Yongquan.

2. Prescription of foot reflecting zones: Point and knead Cerebrum, Neck and Pituitary Gland; push and press from bilateral Accessory Thyroid Gland; point and press bilateral Adrenal Gland; push and press bilaterally from Pelvic Cavity to Genital Gland; and point and press bilateral Celliac Plexus, on the soles. Press from Uterus to Vagina in the medial side of the dorsum of feet, press and knead Ovary on bilateral dorsums of feet at a fixed position. Rotate counterclockwisely the roots of the toes with fingers and pinch and press constantly the bilateral sides of the heels.

Remarks

1. The above point or zone groups are to be massaged twice a day. Continuous application of this therapy is very effective for relieving symptoms of the disease.

2. Patient should live a regular life and have a regular meal, do proper exercises, combine work and rest properly, avoid over fatigue, and keep a pleasant mood.

Emaciation

Emaciation refers to a loss of body weight by 10% or even more than a normal one, which may be caused by a number of factors: ① Heriditary factors, such as family emaciation; ② Diseases of the endocrine system such as hyperthyroidism, diabetes, functional decline of anterior lobe of the pituitary gland, ③ Chronic consumptive diseases, such as chronic infectious diseases, hemopathy and malignant tumours; ④ Diseases of the digestive or respiratory disturbance, such as diseases of the mouth cavity and throat and diseases of the digestive tract; ⑤ Drugs, psychic anorexia and poor appetite due to mental stress.

Essentials of Diagnosis

1. A family history, progressive emaciation, which is constitutional emaciation in most cases, excessive appetite and notable reduce of body weight indicate diabetes and hyperthyroidism; pigmentation of skin or mucosa and poor appetite suggest chronic decline of the adrenocortical function; and long-standing disturbance of digestion and absorption may be seen in chronic pharyngitis or diseases of the esophagus, gastrointestinal tract, liver, gallbladder and pancreas.

2. Emaciation or long-standing low fever with unknown reason may be found in tuberculosis, hyperthyroidism, malignant tumour, etc., and if severe mental disorder is found, it often suggests psychic anorexia.

3. Fall of hair with atrophy of the breast and genitalia is seen in decline of the pituitary gland function; emaciation with polyuria, excessive drinking and excessive eating indicates diabetes; if emaciation is seen in patients with gastrointestinal diseases or chronic liver diseases, it is an emaciation caused by chronic gastrointestinal tract or liver diseases; and the severe emaciation caused by psychic anorexia may present no positive signs other than anorexia.

Massage Treatment

1. Prescription of foot points: Press and knead bilateral Zusanli, Xiajuxu and Sanyinjiao; point and knead bilateral Taixi, Neiting and Gongsun; and rub bilateral Yongquan.

2. Prescription of foot reflecting zones: Press and knead Thyroid Gland in the bilateral soles; push and press Stomach and Duodenum on the bilateral soles; point and press Liver on the right sole; and according to the position of Large Intestine in the soles, push and knead Colon and Small Intestine in the soles in sequence; and push

and press Esophagus in the bilateral soles.
Remarks
1. The above point or zone groups are to be treated twice a day. It is effective for the emaction due to diseases of the digestive tract and psychic anorexia.

2. The symptom may be caused by various causes. So, it is necessary to identify the primary disease and give corresponding treatment to the diseases.

Obesity

When the body weight increases by 20% more than a normal one, it is known as obesity. Fat storage in patient with obesity is obviously greater than the average volume of fat in a healthy person.
Essential of Diagnosis
1. Case history

(1) Obesity with a family history and overweight since childhood is mostly the constitutional obesity; that with a history of over intake of sweat food is an obesity due to excessive eating.

(2) Obesity due to meningitis or cerebral traumatic injury may be seen in interbrain damage; obesity in patients over middle age mostly indicates diabetes; obesity in a woman with amenorrhea or years of sterility may be seen in bilateral polycystic ovary syndrome.

2. Signs

(1) Even obesity may be seen in simple obesity; symmetric obesity suggests Cusine's syndrome; obesity mainly in breast, lower abdomen and perineum with hyposexualism is often seen in adiposogenital dysfunction and is mostly accompanied with immature genetalia.

(2) Obesity complicated by hypertension is seen in Cusine's syndrome or interbrain diseases; that complicated by papill edema or atrophy is often seen in tumours of the hypothalamus or the pituitary gland; and obesity with visual field defect is often seen in acromegalia.

(3) People with increase of body weight are mainly those who take in an energy that exceeds the consumptive capacity of the body from food and as a result, the residual energy is turned into fat and accumulates in the body. Most people with over weight have retarded movements, listlessness, sleepiness, polyhidrosis and hyposexuality.

Massage Treatment

1. Prescription of foot points: Press bilateral Zusanli, Xiajuxu and Sanyinjiao with heavy force; point and knead bilateral Jiexi, Taichong and Neiting; and grasp and knead bilateral Taixi and Kunlun.

2. Prescription of foot reflecting zones: Press and knead bilateral Thyroid Gland, Accessory Thyroid Gland, Pituitary Gland and Esophagus from upper to lower in sequence on the soles; and point and knead Spleen on the left sole.

Remarks

1. The above point or zone groups are to be massaged twice daily, and constant use of this therapy has a better therapeutic effect on ordinary obesity. If such manipulations as kneading, pinching and rubbing are performed on the obesity position, the therapeutic effect will be even better.

2. Patients should control their meal, avoid intake of greasy, fatty or sweat food and keep on physical exercises.

Headache

This is a common and main symptom in many diseases such as angioheadache, ultracranial diseases, intracranial diseases, general diseases, neurosis, neurosism, hysteria and menopausal syndrome.

Essential of Diagnosis

1. Auditory headache due to infection, tumor or obstruction of the auditory tube is mostly localized and unilateral; traumatic headache and headache caused by intracranial or extracranial diseases or extracranial scars is also localized, with a cutaneous pain

and is often induced by excitement or exertion of force; headache due to diseases of the eyes, ears, nose or teeth is often localized and dull in nature; headache caused by acute glaucoma is usually severe and is accompanied with vomiting; headache caused by chronic glaucoma is marked by dull pain in the bilateral foreheads; headache due to diseases of the esophagus, mouth, throat and neck is dull in nature and is not complicated by vomiting; headache due to muscle contraction is related to mental states and is usually located in the bilateral fronto-occipital region or temporal region, with a heaviness sensation, distension and pain in head day and night; headache due to lower pressure in the intracranial cavity is mostly seen in occipital region or vertex, throbbing in nature and is more severe in a standing position, accompanied with nausea and vomiting; headache due to higher pressure of the intracranial cavity, mostly seen in the frontal region or the occipital region, is usually persistent dull pain which is more severe in the morning, usually aggravated by cough or sneeze and is often accompanied with vomiting and visual decline.

2. Vascular headache: This kind of headache is mostly seen in female and usually onsets in the adolescent age, presenting as periodic migraine. It usually attacks in the daytime or in the morning. This condition occurs as a numb sensation in the face, lips and limbs and mild aphasia, then a migraine or headache in the whole head. The pain is usually throbbing dull pain or stabbling pain which is then turned into persistent pain that is accompanied with nuasea, vomiting, constipation, photophobia, congestion of the conjunctiva and nasal mucosa, increased secretion. The attack may last several hours and after the attack, patient feels lassitude and sleepiness. In addition, attack of the headache in female is often related to menstrual period.

3. Acute attack of the headache is usually seen in acute infection, subcutaneous bleeding or after a bone puncture in the lumbar region. Before the attack, patient often experiences restlessness, lassitude, xanthopia, tinnitus, dizziness, yawn with flushing of face, protrudence of vessels in the temporal region or pale in a few cases.

Massage Treatment

1. Prescription of foot points: Press and knead bilateral Yanglingquan and Sanyinjiao; point and knead bilateral Kunlun, Zhaohai and Taichong; pinch and knead bilateral Neiting for cases with pain in the frontal region, bilateral Zulinqi for migraine, bilateral Jinmen for pain in the occipital region and bilateral Yongquan for pain in the vertex.

2. Prescription of foot reflecting zones: Push and press from Cervical Vertebrae to Sacral Vertebrae through the Thoracic Vertebrae and the Lumbar Vertebrae; push and press from Kidney to Bladder through the Ureter in the bilateral soles of feet; pinch and press the Cerebellum, Cervix, Trigerminal Nerve, Temporal Lobe, Cerebrum and Frontal Sinus in the big toes of the feet.

Remarks

1. The above point or zone groups are to be massaged twice a day. This therapy has a better therapeutic effect on headache caused by common cold, neurosism and menopausal syndrome.

2. If the headache fails to be relieved by repeated treatments with this method and it is aggravated further, examinations should be made to see whether there is diseases of the intracranial cavity or not so that the primary disease can be treated in time.

Neurosism

This condition arises from disturbance of the inhibition and excitation of the cerebral cortex due to long-standing mental stress. It is one of the most commonly seen neurosis.

Essential of Diagnosis

1. Attack of the disease is related to long-standing mental stress, seen mostly in the young or the middle aged. It usually has a slow onset and the symptoms vary in severity in different times.

2. It has various kinds of symptoms, such as being extremely sensitive to environment, other people or himself, aversion to sharp light, voice or a mass of people, irritability, distension of head, chest stuffiness, palpitation, abdominal fulness, aching pain of

joints, liability to become tired in both mind and physical strength, forgetfulness, insomnia and dream-disturbed sleep and anxiety; such symptoms of the vegetative nerve and visceral disturbance as tachycardia, hypertension or hypotension, cold or numb limbs, loss of appetite, constipation or diarrhea, frequent urination, irregular menstruation, emission, premature ejaculation or impotence.

Massage Treatment

1. Prescription of foot points: Press and knead bilateral Zusanli and Sanyinjiao; Point and press bilateral Taichong, Zhaohai and Taixi; pinch and press bilateral Xingjian, Yinbai and Lidui; and point and press first and then rub bilateral Yongquan.

2. Prescription of foot reflecting zones: Push, press, pinch and knead Cerebellum, Pituitary Gland, Trigerminal Nerve (Temporal Lobe), Thyroid Gland and Accessory Thyroid Gland on the bilateral soles; push and press from Kidney to Bladder through Ureter on the bilateral soles.

Remarks

1. The above point or zone groups are to be treated twice a day. Constant application of this therapy has a better therapeutic effect on various types of neurosis.

2. This disease is usually inorganic, but similar manifestations may be seen in some organic diseases. So, careful differentiation must be made.

3. Patient should get rid of his or her anxiety, treat the disease in a proper attitude, strengthen his or her confidence in overcoming the disease and keep on physical exercise.

Insomina

This is a common symptom in clinic, which refers to failure to have a normal sleep. It may be caused by many reasons and its pathogenesis is rather complicated. In most cases, it is caused by enhanced nervous sensitivity, over anxiety, emotional upset, over mental stress, terror, or over fatigue and general debility due to long-standing disease. It may also be caused by hypertension, atherosclerosis, infection, sequela of poisoning dysfunction of the gastrointestinal tract, improper diet, injury to the stomach or intestine, retention of food or other diseases.

Essential of Diagnosis

1. Symptoms seen in patients with insomnia: Some patients may fail to fall asleep or fail to fall asleep again after waking up; some may experience frequent wake and sleep or shallow sleep; some may fail to fall asleep all the whole night; and some may fail to sleep and have dream-disturbed sleep.

2. Patients with insomnia often present dizziness, headache, palpitation, forgetfulness, lustreless face, listlessness, lassitude, loose stool, gastric discomfort, dry mouth and throat, irritability, red eyes, bitter taste, or abnormal mental activities or mental states.

Massage Treatment

1. Prescriptions of foot points: Press and knead bilateral Zusanli and Sanyinjiao; point and knead bilateral Taixi, Zhaohai and Shenmai; press energically bilateral Taichong, Gongsun and Neiting; pinch and press bilateral Shimian, Yinbai and Lidui; and rub bilateral Yongquan until a hot sensation is produced.

2. Prescription of foot reflecting zones: Push and press Pelvic Cavity in the soles; pinch, press, push and knead the Cerebrum, Frontal Sinus, Temporal Lobe, Cerebellum, Cerebral Pituitary Gland, Thyroid Gland and Celliac Plexus from the upper to the lower; push and press from Kidney to Bladder through Ureter; Push and press Liver in the right sole and Spleen in the left sole.

Remarks

1. The above point or zone groups are to be treated twice a day. Constant application of this therapy has a better therapeutic effect on the disease.

2. During the treatment, patient should keep a stable mood, avoid smoking, drinking strong tea or coffee before sleep and take part in proper physical exercise.

Trigerminal Neuralgia

This refers to paroxysmal transient sharp pain that frequently occurs in the zone where the trigeriminal nerve is distributed. It usually has not the manifestations of disturbance of nerve conduction such as anesthesia and is mostly seen in people over 40 years old. It affects female more than male, is usually unilateral and mostly involves the second and the third branches of the trigeminal nerve.

Essential of Diagnosis

1. Sudden onset with an electric shock, burning, prickling or sting sensation in the affected part, convulsion of the facial muscles, conjunctiva congestion, skin flushing, chewing, lacrimation or salivation in the affected side. Such patients often rub or knead the affected part to relieve the pain which may last several seconds or several minutes. In the remission stage, there is not any discomfort.

2. The pain is usually induced by speaking, chewing, washing face, teeth-brushing, exposure to cold or touching a point in the face, with a tendency to be aggravated day by day.

3. Examinations on the nervous system show no sensory or motor disturbance.

Massage Treatment

1. Prescription of the foot points: Point and knead bilateral Yongquan; knead heavily bilateral Neiting and Jiexi on the dorsum of feet and Kunlun near the malleoluses of the feet; pinch and press bilateral Bafeng on the dorsum of feet; and push heavily the metatarsal spaces and the metatarso-phlangeal articulations.

2. Pescription of the foot reflecting zones: Knead and pinch bilateral Trigerminal Nerve and Temporal Lobe with a strong force; push and press bilateral cerebrum, Neck and Eyes from the upper to the lower; and press and knead bilaterals Accessory Thyroid Gland in the soles and Cervical Vetebrae in the medial side of the dorsum of feet at fixed positions.

Remarks

1. The above points or zone groups are to be treated twice a day. This treatment is very effective for primary trigerminal neuralgia.

2. Causes of the secondary trigerminal neuralgia should be identified in order to give corresponding treatment.

Epilepsy

This is a syndrome caused by repeated electric shock of the neuron which gives rise to transient and sudden cerebral dysfunction. It has two types, the primary and the secondary, and the disease may be caused by congenital brain defect. Meningitis, brain tumors, cerebral parositosis, hypertension, cerebral atherosclerosis, traumatic injury to the brain or gestosis can all lead to secondary epilepsy, while the primary epilepsy, which may be related to inheridity, is mostly seen in the young below 20 years old.

Essential of Diagnosis

1. Grant mal epilepsy: This is characterized by loss of consciousness and general convulsion. Most of the primary epilepsy have not premonitoring symptoms. Patients tend to have muscular tonics at a movement and then fall with consequent loss of consciousness and general convulsion. The secondary epilepsy usually starts with local symptoms. When bilateral convulsion develops, patients have loss of consciousness with myotonic contraction, upward staring of eyes, platycoria, light reflex disappearance, sweating, tenesmus, salivation, laryngeal tetanus with shouting, apnea and purplish face. Then, this condition is turned into intermittent tetanus with white or bloody foam, incontinence of defecation and urination or vomiting. At last, the tetanus stops suddenly and the patients come to their mind gradually which is followed by lethargy. When patients fully restore to their normal mind, they still have headache, general pain, lassitude and remember nothing about the seizure. If the great seizure happens repeatedly with failure of the consciousness to be restored, it suggests a status epilepticus, which is often accompanied with high fever, dehydration and cerebral edema, and

may lead to death as a result of respiratory or circulatory failure.

2. Minor epilepsy: Seen mostly in children or the adolescence, this condition is marked by temporary disturbance of consciousness without general tetanus, sudden stoppage of activity in which patients show no response, staring or up staring of eyes, or by short and rapid muscular tetanus which restores to normal at a movement. Patients remember nothing about the seizure and this condition occurs frequently.

3. Localized epilepsy: Motor attack is manifested as localized tetanus, transient aphonia, turning of head and eyes toward one side, etc., the sensory attack is marked by localized sensory abnormality, special tasting or smelling, and the visceral attack is symptomized as salivation, vomiting, abdominal pain, palpitation, dyspnea, incontinence of urine, headache, etc.

4. Psychomotor attack: This condition exhibits temporary mental symptoms and loss of consciousness, accompanied with emotional changes as terror, depression and forced thinking. On attack, patients have a vague mind, repeat one posture mechanically or do involuntary act, speak simple words, shout or sing. After the attack, consciousness is restored and patients remember nothing about the attack.

Massage Treatment

1. Prescription of foot points: Press and knead bilateral Sanyinjiao; point and knead bilateral Shenmai, Zhaohai and Taichong; pinch and knead bilateral Neiting, Pushen, Jinmen, Gongsun and Yongquan.

2. Prescription of foot reflecting zones: Pinch and knead Cerebrum on the soles; push and press Lympthatic Gland of Upper Body, the Lymph Gland of Lower Body and the Lymph Gland of the Thorax on the dorsum of feet.

Remarks

1. The above point or zone groups are to be treated twice a day with moderate stimuli in ordinary days and heavy stimuli during the attack. Long-standing application of this therapy has the effect of reducing the frequency of attack and relieving the symptoms in the

attack.

2. Causes of the secondary epilepsy must be identified first with corresponding examinations so as to give corresponding treatment to the primary diseases.

Hysteria

This is a morbid condition marked by paroxysmal phrenoblabia and bodily disturbance induced by mental disorders or unfavorable hint, which is mostly seen in young female. It has an acute attack and a short illness course, and will be relieved quickly in the case of proper hint being given.

Essential of Diagnosis

1. Phrenoblabia: This is marked by emotional burstout, sudden occurrence of mental confusion, vague consciousness, crying, laughing or arguing without reason, dance for joy or even fantastic acts, and burstout of unhappiness without limitation. Patients can remember the process after the attack clearly.

2. Bodily disturbance: This is manifested as hysteric paralysis, hysteric aphonia, hysteric tetanus, etc. The hysteric paralysis is usually marked by tonic paralysis in the upper or lower limb of one side, or relaxant paralysis in a few cases which may restore to normal in a short time. It may also be manifested as excessive act which lasts a longer time, marked by restlessness of the limbs, shouting, incontinence of urine and foamy spittle during the attack. The attack is rarely seen during sleep.

3. Anesthesia or oversensitivity in some aspects: They may have sudden deafness, blindness or aphonia, but they can go around an obstacle and may turn back when some sounds are produced in their side or behind them. Besides, such symptoms of vegetative nerve as vomiting, hiccup, palpitation and shortness of breath may present.

Massage Treatment

1. Prescription of the foot points: Press and knead bilateral Zusanli and Sanyinjiao; point and knead bilateral Fenglong and Gong-

sun; pinch and knead bilateral Zhongchong and Yongquan. For cases with hysteric deafness, point and knead bilateral Xiaxi, and pinch and knead bilateral Zuqiaoyin additionally; for cases with hysteric amaurosis, point and knead bilateral Taichong, Xingjian and Guangming additionally; for cases with hysteric aphonia, point and knead Taixi and Zhaohai additionally; and for cases with hysteric paralysis, press and point bilateral Weizhong, Chengshan, Feiyang and Yanglingquan heavily.

2. Prescription of foot reflecting zone: Push and press Head (Cerebrum), Frontal Sinus, Brain Stem and Cerebellum on the soles of feet.

Remarks

1. The above point or zone groups are to be treated twice a day. If hint therapy is also adopted simultaneously, it has a remarkabale therapeutic effect.

2. This disease usually shows no positive result in ordinary physical examinations or laboratory test, and it should be distinguished from organic diseases of the nervous system.

3. Patients should be actively encouraged to strengthen their confidence in overcoming the disease. Their anxiety must be removed so that they can keep a calm mind to receive corresponding treatment.

Facial Paralysis

This disease refers to peripheral facial paralysis caused by acute non-pyogenic facial neuritis, which may be related to viral infection, allergic reaction or inadequate blood supply.

Essential of Diagnosis

1. This disease may affect the population of any age and before occurrence of the disease, there is usually acute pharygeal infection due to attack of cold wind. It onsets suddenly and is usually noticed when getting up in the morning or when brushing one's teeth or washing one's face in the morning.

2. It usually attacks the facial nerve of one side. Initially, it ex-

hibits pain in the ear, mastoid process or the mandibles, then, there is paralysis of the expression muscles, disappearance of the wrinkles, expansion of the eye width, exposure of sclera, tearing, shallowing of the nasolabial groove, ptosis of the mouth corner, salivation, failure to do such movements as knitting one's forehead and brows, shutting eyes or expanding one's cheeks. When teeth are exposed, the mouth corner inclines toward the healthy side.

3. This disease usually begins to be recovered 2～3 weeks after its onset and may restore to normal in 1～6 months. A few cases who fail to recover from the disease may develop convulsion, contracture or synkinesia of the facial muscles.

Massage Treatment

1. Prescription of the foot points: Press and knead bilateral Zusanli and Sanyinjiao; point and knead bilateral Neiting, Xiaxi, Taichong and Chongyang; and pinch and press bilateral Lidui.

2. Prescription of foot reflecting zones: Press and knead Cerebrum, Eyes, Nose, Trigerminal Nerve, Temporal Lobe and Front Sinus on the soles of feet.

Remarks

1. The above point or zone groups are to be treated twice a day. Combined use of this therapy and facial massage and hot compress on the face can bring about better therapeutic effects.

2. At the early stage of the disease, the stimuli should not be too strong. Manipulations should be strengthened 3 weeks later gradually. During the treatment, patients should be kept away from wind or cold.

3. This disease should be distinguished from central facial paralysis and the space-occupying lesions in the intracranial cavity.

Sciatica

This is a disease caused by diseases of the sciatic nerve or its adjacent tissues.

Essential of Diagnosis

1. More than 90% of sciatica are caused by herniatid disk, with a history of over loading or traumatic injury of the lumbar region.

2. It attacks suddenly, starting with pain in the lumbar region which then radiates downward along the hip, posterior aspect of the thigh and the lower leg rapidly. It is often aggravated by walk, cough, sneezing, or turning body.

3. In a standing position, the loin inclines to the diseased side or the healthy side with a bit reflexion of the affected limb, tenderness beside the lumbar vertebrae which radiates to the lower leg.

4. There is weakening of the strength of dorsal reflexion of the toe in the affected side, sensory numbness or retardation of skin in the lateral side of the lower leg and the dorsum of foot, and muscular atrophy of the affected leg in the later stage.

Massage Treatment

1. Prescription of foot points: Press and knead bilateral Weizhong, Yanglingquan and Zusanli; point and knead Chengshan, Juegu, Kunlun and Qiuxu; knead heavily and point and press bilateral Taichong, Jinggu and Zulinqi; and pinch and knead bilateral Yongquan.

2. Prescription of foot reflecting zones: Push and press from Kidney to Bladder through Ureter on the soles of feet; pinch, knead, press and push bilateral Sciatic Nerve; press and knead Hip Joint in the lateral sides of the dorsal sides of the feet and the femur on the medial sides of the feet.

Remarks

1. The above point or zone groups are to be treated twice a day with emphasis placed on the affected side. Constant application of this therapy has a better therapeutic effect.

2. This is a symptom caused by many kinds of diseases, so a definite diagnosis must be made. If it is caused by tumor or tuberculosis, the primary diseases should be treated. If it is caused by herniated disk, Tuina therapy shoud be employed simultaneously in order to achieve an even better effect.

3. Patients with severe pain at the acute stage should be kept in bed for rest. When the symptom is relieved, they should do proper

activities or exercises and keep themselves warm.

Surgical Diseases

Appendicitis

This is one of the most commonly seen surgical diseases of the abdomen, which is an acute abdominal disease caused by obstruction of the appendicular cavity and suprainfection of multiple bacteria. The obstruction is mostly caused by faeces, stone, foreign body, round worm or eggs of the round wrom, or adhesion, distortion, or proliferation of the lymphatic tissues; while the infection mostly arises from the obstruction which leads to inadequate blood supply to the appendix, reproduction of bacteria in the tract, spread of the inflammation of the adjacent tissues and the ensuing lymphatic infection.

Essential of Diagnosis

1. Acute appendicitis: This condition has a sudden onset, manifested as pain in the upper abdomen or around the umbilicus which then shifts to the right lower abdomen several hours later. The pain is persistent and aggravated paroxysmally, and such accompanying symptoms as nausea, vomiting, poor appetite, constipation, diarrhea or fever are often presented. In the right lower abdomen, there is notable tenderness or even rebouncing tenderness and guarding of the abdominal muscles in severe cases.

2. Chronic appendicitis: Repeated or persistent dull pain in the right lower abdomen which is often induced or aggravated by violent activity, overwalking and improper diet and may be accompanied with distending pain in the upper abdomen, constipation or increase of frequence of defecation, localized tenderness in the appendix region of the right lower abdomen, mild guarding of the abdominal muscles or nodular-like mass palpated sometimes.

Massage Treatment

1. Prescription of foot points: Point and knead bilateral Zusanli

and Lanweixue; press heavily bilateral Neiting, Taichong, Taibai and Gongsun.

2. Prescription of foot reflecting zones: Push and press Stomach and Duodenum in the soles of the feet; push and press inward Cecum and Appendix; and push and press bilateral Lymph Gland of the Lower Body of the feet from upper to lower.

Remarks

1. The above point or zone groups are to be treated twice a day. It has a better effect for simple acute appendicitis.

2. Patients with a tendency of perforation or necrosis should be treated with surgical means in time.

Haemorrhoids

This refers to the venous masses caused by expansion and varicosis of venous plexus of anal canal. The haemorrhoid with a surface of mucous membrane is called internal haemorrhoid, that with a surface of skin is termed external haemorrhoid, and that with both the internal haemorrhoid and the external haemorrhoid is called mixed haemorrhoid.

Essential of Diagnosis

1. External haemorrhoid: At the initial stage, the skin around the anus prominents circularly without notable symptoms. When rupture of the veins and thrombopoiesis in the external haemorrhoid develop, there is severe swelling and pain which is aggravated by defecation, walk or sitting. In the subcutaneous region of the anal border, there is prominent blue or purple masses.

2. Internal heamorrhoid: At stage I, there is bleeding with bright blood, no pain, separated faeces and blood which may be either only several drops in volume in mild cases or even projectile in nature in severe cases in defecation. The bleeding usually stops after defecation and the haemorrhoid core doesn't protrude out of the anus. At stage II, the haemorrhoid core protrudes out of the anus in defecation but can retract itself after the defecation. The mucous mem-

brane is thickened and bleeding is reduced. At stage III, the protruded haemorrhoid core cannot retract itself and it may protrude even in the case of walking or coughing. The pain is aggravated when infection, erosion or incarceration of the haemorrhoid core occurs.

3. Mixed haemorrhoid: This condition has the features of both the internal haemorrhoid and the external haemorrhoid and is relatively severe in illness condition.

Massage Treatment

1. Prescription of foot points: Press and knead bilateral Chengshan and Feiyang; point and knead bilateral Ludisanzhen; pinch and knead bilateral Shugu and Yongquan.

2. Prescription of foot reflecting zones: Push and press bilaterally from Adrenal Gland to Bladder through Kidney and Ureter; push and press from Sigmoid to Anus through Rectum in the left sole; push upward by grasping Rectum and Anus in the medial sides of feet behind the malleoluses; and push and press Lymph Gland of the Upper Body and Lymph Gland of Lower Body on the dorsal side of the feet.

Remarks

1. The above point or zone groups are to be treated twice a day. If pressing and kneading the tip of the tail bone clockwise and counterclockwise for 30~50 times each respectively is adopted simultaneously, the therapeutic effect will be even better.

2. Patients should avoid over fatigue, standing long, having heavy loading or eating pungent and acrid food and keep their defecation smooth.

Periarthritis of the Shoulder

This is a disease marked by chronic inflammation and degenerative diseases of such soft tissues as muscles, tendons and joint capsules around the shoulder joint, which affects more frequently the middle aged or the aged. Most patients have a history of exposure to cold, traumatic injury or chronic strain of the shoulder.

Essential of Diagnosis

1. Rigidity of shoulder with aversion to cold, wide soreness or cutting pain which is mild in the daytime and severe at night and radiates to the neck and the upper arms. The disease may last several weeks, several months or even several years.

2. Limited abduction, extorsion, dorsiflexion and lifting of the shoulder joint, or even inability to comb one's hair, put on one's cloth or tie the waist belt. In severe cases, the movements of the shoulder joint may disappear completely, or rigid shoulder may develop.

3. In the acute stage, there is sharp pain on touching, while in the chronic stage, there exists wide tenderness with fixed painful point on percussion sometimes.

Massage Treatment

1. Prescription of foot points: Press and knead bilateral Yinlingquan, Zusanli and Sanyinjiao; point and knead bilateral Chengshan; and pinch and knead bilateral Tiaokou and Taichong.

2. Prescription of foot reflecting zones: Push and press Shoulder in the soles from upper to lower and Trapezius Muscle from the medial side to the lateral side; press Accessory Thyroid Gland in the soles; point and knead Cervical Vertebrae in the medial side of the dorsum of feet; push and press Shoulder and Scapula in the lateral side of the dorsum of feet from the anterior side to the posterior side and the bilateral Lymph Gland of Upper Body in the dorsum of feet.

Remarks

1. The above point or zone groups are to be treated twice a day. During the treatment, more strengthen should be exerted and the patient should be ordered to do such movements of shoulder as lifting, backward extension and abduction so as to achieve better therapeutic effect.

2. The primary diseases must be identified clearly. Foot massage therapy is not effective for the periarthritis of shoulder caused by tuberculosis or tumor, and the primary diseases must be treated in time.

3. Patients should keep their shoulders warm in ordinary days. Besides, they should do proper functional exercise to prevent adhension of the joint.

Cervical Spondopathy

This is a syndrome caused by degenerative disorders of the intravertebral dics or hyperosteogeny of the cervical vertebrae which presses the cervical nervous root, cervical artery, sympathetic nerve or the spinal cord. It has a slow onset, and is mostly seen in the population over 40 years old. Damage of such tissues as intravertebral dics and ligaments due to various kinds of acute or chronic traumatic injuries serves as external cause of the disease, while degenerative disorders of the intravertebral dics and hyperosteogeny of the cervical vertebrae, which give rise to inflammation, stimuli and press of the cervical nervous root, serve as the internal causes of the disease.

Essential of Diagnosis

1. Cervical spondopathy of venous root type: This is marked by persistent pain in the shoulder and neck, which often radiates to the upper limb of one side or bilateral sides. The pain is mostly stabbing pain in nature which is usually more severe at night or aggravated by backward extension of the neck or cough and relieved by lying flat, elevating shoulder and flexing elbow. When the 6th cervical nervous root is pressed, there is stabbing pain and numbness in the thumb, weakening or disappearance of the biceps reflex; when the 7th cervical nervous root is pressed, there is stabbing pain and numbness in the index finger and the middle finger; and when the 8th cervical nervous root is pressed, there is stabbling pain and numbness in the ring finger and the little finger.

2. Cervical spondopathy of spinal cord type: When the spinal cord is pressed, there is numbness of the lower limbs in the early stage which is then followed by numbness of the upper limbs, failure to grasp firmly or even paralysis of the limbs. Besides, there is

weakneing of the sensation in the trunk and lower limbs, tendon hyperreflexia, increased muscular tension, or even contracture of the ankles with inability to stand.

3. Cervical spondopathy of the vertebral artery type: This type is marked by pain in the neck, shoulder and occipital region, dizziness, nausea, vomiting, positional vertigo, sudden fall, failure to hold things, tinnitus, deafness and blurred vision, which are often induced or aggravated by turning head or bending aside to a certain position.

4. Cervical spondopathy of sympathetic type: This is a condition marked by pain in the occipital region, heaviness of the head, dizziness or migraine, palpitation, chest stuffiness, cold limbs, cold skin or feverish sensation in the hands and feet and soreness of the limbs due to stimuli to the sympathetic nerve.

5. Mixed cervical spondopathy: When symptoms of two or even more of the above mentioned types coexist, it is a mixed cervical spondopathy which is the most commonly seen type in the clinic.

Massage Treatment
1. Prescription of foot points

Nervous root type: Press and knead bilateral Yanglingquan and Juegu; point and knead Waiqiu and Kunlun in the lateral side of feet; and pinch and knead bilateral Tiaokou, Jinmen and Shugu.

Spinal cord type: Press and knead bilateral Weizhong, Chengshan and Sanyinjiao; point and knead bilateral Feiyang and Chengjin; and pinch and knead bilateral Taichong, Neiting, Qiuxu, Shangqiu and Yongquan.

Cervical artery type: Press and knead bilateral Zusanli and Sanyinjiao; point and knead bilateral Zhaohai, Taixi and Taichong; and pinch and knead bilateral Yongquan.

Sympathetic type: Press and knead bilateral Zusanli, Sanyinjiao and Fuyang; point and knead bilateral Guangming, Xiaxi and Taichong; and pinch, knead and rub bilateral Yongquan.

2. Prescription of foot reflecting zones: Knead Head, Neck, Trapezius Muscle and Accessory Thyroid Gland in the soles; push and press Liver in the right sole; point and press bilateral Kidney in

the soles; push and press from Cervical Vertebrae to Thoracic Vertebrae through Accessory Thyroid Gland in the medial side of the dorsum of feet.

Remarks

1. The above point or zone groups are to be treated twice a day. Constant application of this therapy has a better therapeutic effect on all types of cervical spondopathy. For the mixed type, points or zones should be formulated based on the prescriptions for the different types according to clinical manifestations.

2. Patients shouldn't sleep on a pillow with a big height and should do proper functional exercise such as forward bending, backward extension, side extension, side rotation or circular rotation. If cervical tracting is used in combination, the therapeutic effect will be even better.

Stiff Neck

This is a disease marked by acute rigidity and pain of the neck and nape with limited movement, which is mostly caused by improper body posture in sleeping or sleeping on a high pillow with sprain, contusion and exposure to cold or wind.

Essential of Diagnosis

1. Rigidity and pain of the neck and nape, which often radiates to the shoulder and the upper limbs. The head inclines to the affected side while the lower jaw inclines to the healthy side. When patient tries to turn his neck, his body often has to be turned together.

2. Increased tension and tenderness in the cervical muscles of the diseased side which is most severe in the inner angle of the scapula, with movement limitation.

Massage Treatment

1. Prescription of the foot points: Press and knead bilateral Yanglingquan; point and knead bilateral Juegu and Kunlun; knead bilateral Qiuxu and Neiting heavily; and pinch and knead Shugu.

2. Prescription of the foot reflecting zones: Pinch and knead Neck

in the soles; push and press Trapezius Muscle and Shoulder; and press and knead Cervical Vertebrae in the medial side of feet from the upper to the lower.

Remarks

1. The above point or zone groups are to be massaged twice a day. In the treatment, order the patient to slightly and gently turn his neck. When the pain is relieved, patient may extend the movements.

2. Keep the neck warm and avoid using high pillow.

Emission

This refers to frequent ejaculations in the case of absence of sexual intercourse.

Essential of Diagnosis

1. It is considered normal if an adult unmarried man or a man who doesn't not live together with his wife has one or twice emissions a month. However, it will be a morbid condition if two or even more emissions occur a week or emission occurs in a clear mind.

2. Most patients have such accompanying symptoms as soreness of loins, aching in the back, dizziness, tinnitus, lassitude and listlessness. Following an emission during sleep, there is usually flushed face, bitter taste in the mouth, vexation and dark urine. If the emission happens unconsciously in the sleep, patient may present a dull eyesight, listlessness or secondary emission on thinking about sex, emaciation, sweating, dizziness and decline of memory.

Massage Treatment

1. Prescription of foot points: Press and knead bilateral Ququan and Sanyinjiao; knead heavily bilateral Fuliu, Taixi and Zhaohai; and pinch, knead and rub bilateral Yongquan.

2. Rub soles with more strength, twist the big toes and massage the heels.

3. Push and press Adrenal Gland and Kidney in the soles; push and press bilateral Thyroid Gland and Heart in the left sole from the

lower to the upper; press the bilateral Pituitary Gland in the soles at a fixed position; and press Genital Gland in the soles.

Remarks

1. The above points and reflecting zones are to be massaged twice a day. If rubbing Yaoyan up and down with palms for 30~50 times is adopted also in each treatment, the therapeutic effect will be even better.

2. The disease should be explained carefully to the patient so that he can get rid of his worries and treat the diseases correctly.

3. The primary diseases must be treated simultaneously if the emission is caused by some organic diseases.

Prostatitis

This is a disease caused by infection of staphylococcus or streptococcus, which can be classified as the acute and the chronic. Patients used to have such induction factors as overdrinking, improper sexual life, traumatic injury of the perineum, common cold or acute urethritis before suffering from the disease.

Essential of Diagnosis

1. Acute prostatitis: This is marked by acute onset with high fever, chills, frequent, urgent and painful urination, occasional glossary hematuria, distending pain or severe pain in the sacral region or perineum.

2. Chronic prostatitis: This type has a slow onset and is usually secondary to the acute prostatitis. It is manifested as mild frequent urination with a burning sensation during the urination and drippling in the end of the urination. The terminal urine is turbid, and white secretion is often detected in the opening of the urethra. In addition, there is lowering-down sensation in the lumbo-sacral region, perineum or scrotum. Some patients may also have manifestations of sexual disorder as impotence or pain in ejaculation or neurosism.

Massage Treatment

1. Prescription of foot points: Press and knead bilateral Ququan,

Zusanli and Sanyinjiao; point and knead bilateral Taixi, Zhaohai, Taichong and Kunlun; pinch and knead bilateral Gongsun and Yongquan.

2. Prescription of foot reflecting zones: Push and press Genital Gland in the soles, then push and knead from Kidney to Bladder through Ureter; press and knead bilateral Pituitary Gland at a fixed position; push and press Heart in the left sole and Liver in the right sole; grasp and push Prostate Gland in the medial side of the dorsum of feet from lower to upper; and massage Lymph Gland of Lower Body from upper to lower.

Remarks

1. The above point or zone groups are to be treated twice a day. Long-standing application of this therapy has a better therapeutic effect on chronic prostatitis.

2. Surgical measures should be given in time to the patients with acute prostatitis marked by general poisoning symptoms such as high fever, hematuria, emission with blood or severe abdominal pain.

Acute Lumbar Sprain

This is one of the commonly seen surgical disease, which is caused by bearing unbearable gravitis or rotating force which gives rise to injury of the tissues in the lumbar region. In this case, lumbar muscles and ligament may undergo sprain as a result of imbalanced exertion of force in the bilateral sides of the loin in the case of improper posture, bending to pick a heavy artical, shouldering or lifting the weights. Sprain of lumbar muscles, ligaments and tendons may also develop when the muscles contracts excessively in the case of exertion of force or exercise without adequate preparations.

Essential of Diagnosis

1. At the movement of the sprain, there is a shock or broken feeling in the lumbar region, severe pain and inability to move. The

pain is often aggravated by cough and may become even severe after staying in bed or on the second day following the strain.

2. In a standing position, patient often supports his waist with his hands. There is rigidity of the lumbar muscles with limited movement and marked tenderness. The painful points vary with the portions affected. Injury of muscle or tendon may exhibit a painful point in one side or bilateral sides of the spinal column and may start half a day later or on the second day after the sprain, and the pain is aggravated gradually.

3. The movement of loin is limited. The pain is relatively mild in rest and aggravated by exercise or cough. There is rigidity of the muscles in the local zone with tenderness and remarkable tracting pain but vibrating pain is absent. Some patients may have radiating pain in the lower limbs. If it is a contusion, hematoma may be noticed in the affected part.

Massage Treatment

1. Prescription of foot points: Press and knead bilateral Weizhong and Yanglingquan; point and knead bilateral Juegu, Kunlun and Chengshan; rub heavily bilateral heels and Taichong.

2. Prescription of foot reflecting zone: Push constantly from Adrenal Gland to the Kidney in the soles; push and knead Liver in the left sole; press and knead at fixed positions Lymph Gland of the Upper Body and Lymph Gland of the Lower Body; and push and press Back Vertebrae, Lumbar Vertebrae and the Inner Tail Bone in the medial side of the feet back and fro. In addition, push and knead the medial border of the soles and the lower end of the sublaxation of talus in the dorsum.

Remarks

1. The above point or zone groups are to be treated twice a day. If the painful point in the affected part is also massaged 30~50 times in each treatment, the therapeutic effect will be even better.

2. Patient should have a proper rest during the treatment so that the lumbar muslces can be relaxed and the sprain be relieved sooner.

Impotence

This refers to failure of the penis to erect or erect hard and the ensuing inability to complete a sexual intercourse although he still has the sexual desire. It is a kind of troublesome sexual disorder in man, which may be caused by such organic diseases of the reproductive organs as deformity of the penis or traumatic injury to the nerves. In most cases, however, it is caused by strengthened inhibition of the brain cortex to the erection and dysfunction of the spinal cord due to such emotional disorders as over nervousness and listlessness, over fatigue, chronic lumbago or a history of masturbation in child age.

Essential of Diagnosis

1. Occasional impotence in a healthy man due to over fatigue, excessive drinking, etc. shouldn't be considered to be a morbid state. Only long-standing repeated occurrence of impotence suggests a morbid state.

2. Most impotence patients have dizziness, vertigo, lassitude, listlessness, insomnia, cold sweating, sallow complexion, restlessless, poor appetite and soreness of loins.

Massage Treatment

1. Prescription of foot points: Press and knead bilateral Zusanli, Ququan and Yingu; point and knead bilateral Sanyinjiao, Taixi and Fuliu; pinch and knead bilateral Taichong and Zhongfeng; and pinch, knead and rub bilateral Yongquan until a hot sensation is produced there.

2. Prescription of foot reflecting zones: Push and press from Kidney to Bladder through Ureter in the soles; push and press Genital Gland in the soles; grasp and push Prostate Gland, Ureter and Genital Gland on the dorsum of feet from lower to upper and Inguinal Groove from upper to lower; point and press Pituitary Gland in the soles of feet; press and knead Heart and Spleen in the left sole; knead digitally Liver in the right sole toward the heel.

Remarks

1. The above point or zone groups are to be treated twice a day. If rubbing the lower abdomen clockwise and counterclockwise respectively for 30~50 times and rubbing Yaoyan with palms up and down for 30~50 times are also adopted, the therapeutic effect will be even better.

2. This disease is a functional sexual disorder. In the treatment, doctor should explain the condition to the patient so that he can get rid of his worries and treat the treatment properly.

3. Treatment must be aimed at the primary diseases if the impotence is caused by organic diseases.

Male Sterility

This refers to sterility in a couple who live together for more than 3 years after marriage due to disorders of the husband.

Essential of Diagnosis

1. Failure to give birth to child in a couple who live together for more than 3 years after marriage and no abnormality of the wife is revealed.

2. Most patients have cryptorchidism, scrotitis secondary to parotitis, prostatitis, seminal vesiculography, epididymitis, uthritis, tuberculosis of the reproductive system, varicocele spermophebectasia, severe hypospadia and a history of traumatic injury, vitamin deficiency, disorder of endocrine system or severe chronic diseases.

3. Clear and thin sperma or inadequate activity of the sperm, disturbance of the sperm-generation function of the testis and sexual disturbance can cause failure of the sperma to combine with a normal ovary cell to result in a conception.

Massage Treatment

1. Prescription of foot points: Press and knead bilateral Zusanli, Ququan and Yingu; knead digitally bilateral Sanyinjiao, Zhaohai and Fuliu; press heavily bilateral Taichong and Taixi; and rub bilateral Yongquan until a hot sensation is produced.

2. Prescription of foot reflecting zones: Push and press bilateral Adrenal Gland and Kidney in the soles; press and knead bilateral Genital Gland in the soles; pinch and knead Pituitary Glands on the big toes of feet; point and knead Heart and Spleen in the left sole; and knead Liver in the right sole digitally from the toes toward the heel.

Remarks

1. The above point or zone groups are to be treated twice a day. If rubbing lower abdomen clockwise and counterclockwise respectively for 30~50 times and rubbing testis for 30~50 times are also adopted in the treatment, the therapeutic effects will be even better.

2. For cases with organic diseases such as hypospadia, tuberculosis and prostatitis, the treatment should be aimed actively at the primary diseases.

Pediatric Diseases

Infantile Indigestion

This is a syndrome caused by non-infectious diseases of the intestine or unknown diseases. Fundamentally, its causes can be generalized as infection out of the intestinal tract, excessive, inadequate or irregular eating, exposure to cold or summer heat, improper care, or allergic to milk or other supplementary foods.

Essential of Diagnosis

1. Presence of manifestations of infection out of the intestine or other pathogenic factors.

2. Mild gastrointestinal symptoms, watery or loose stool which is yellow or yellow-green in color or with some mucous fluid, several or more than a dozen of defecations a day.

3. Poor appetite, abdominal fullness, insomnia, fever in a few cases, vomiting with undigested food, absence of dehydration or acidosis.

Massage Treatment

1. Prescription of foot points: Press and knead bilateral Zusanli, Yinlingquan, Shangjuxu and Xiajuxu; point and knead bilateral Neiting and Gongsun; pinch and knead bilateral Taichong, Taibai and Lineiting; and press digitally and rub bilateral Yongquan toward the right.

2. Prescription of the foot reflecting zones: Push and press Stomach, Duodenum and Pancreas in the soles; massage bilateral Small Intestine from the upper to the lower; point and knead Spleen in the left sole; and push and press Lymph Gland of the Upper Body and the Lymph Gland of the Lower Body in the dorsum of the feet from upper to lower.

Remarks

1. The above point or zone groups are to be treated twice a day. It will bring about remarkable therapeutic effect if it is applied in combination with rubbing the umbilicus with plam clockwise and counterclockwise for 30~50 times respectively.

2. Cases with manifestations of such severe conditions as dehydration and acidosis should be treated by using combined Chinese and Western medicine.

Epidemic Parotitis

This is an acute infectious disease caused by mumps virus which is affected by foams. It occurs mostly in winter and mainly affects the children of 5~9 years old. One may develop a life-long immunity to the disease following the infection.

Essential of Diagnosis

1. A history of contacting with mumps patients and a 2~3 weeks of incubation period.

2. It onsets suddenly, manifested as mild headache and general discomfort initially, which are followed 1~2 days later by swelling of the parotid gland of one side and then the other side. The swelling takes the ear lobe as its center and is diffusive without a clear margin. It is mildly painful on pressing and is elastic. The skin

is not red and the pain is aggravated when chewing or eating acid food. In the cheeks, the opening of the parotid gland is red and swollen, and submanidibular gland and sublinguial gland may also present swelling. Patients have sore throat, poor appetite, vomiting, fever and other general symptoms become more obvious. The disease lasts about 7~12 days.

Massage Treatment

1. Prescription of foot points: Press and knead Sanyinjiao and Ququan; point and knead bilateral Taichong, Xingjian and Xiaxi; pinch and knead bilateral Lidui and Zuqiaoyin; and point and press bilateral Yongquan.

2. Prescription of foot reflecting zones: Press and knead from Kidney to Bladder through Ureter in the soles of feet; press and knead Cerebrum and Frontal Sinus in the soles; push and knead Trigerminal Nerve and Temporal Lobe from upper to lower; push and press Lymph Gland of Upper Body from upper to lower at fixed point; press and knead toe by toe the Lymph Gland of the Whole Body; and press Inguinal Groove for male child complicated with testitis additionally.

Remarks

1. The above point or zone groups are to be treated twice a day. This therapy has a better therapeutic effect on the disease.

2. This disease is infectious, so proper isolation measures should be taken. Besides, other therapies should be adopted in combination for cases with severe complications.

Infantile Anorexia

This is also a common pediatric disease.

Essential of Diagnosis

No appetite, sallow face, emaciation, withering and gradually developed bundling of hair, imbalance of nutrition due to improper diet or preference for certain food, abdominal knuckle, listlessness, etc.

Massage Treatment

1. Prescription of foot points: Press and knead bilateral Zusanli and Xiajuxu; point and knead bilateral Neiting, Taichong and Gongsun; and pinch and knead bilateral Taibai and Lidui on the feet.

2. Prescriptions of foot reflecting zones: Push and press bilateral Stomach, Duodenum and Pancreas in the soles; point and press Spleen in the left sole; push and press Small Intestine in the bilateral soles; and push and press continuously from Kidney to Bladder through Ureter.

Remarks

1. The above point or zone groups are to be treated twice a day. The therapeutic effect will be even better if rubbing abdomen clockwise for 30~50 times in each treatment is also adopted.

2. Ask for the children to have a proper meal or have meals in proper amount at regular times and avoid eating cold, raw, greasy or too sweat food.

Gynecological Diseases

Irregular Menstruation

Irregular menstruation, a common gynecological disease, refers to abnormal changes of the menstruation in period, color, amount and quality. Menstruation is a regular uterine bleeding under the regulation of anterior lobe of the pituitary gland and the hormones secreted from ovary. Thus, disturbance of the anterior lobe of the pituitary gland and the ovary will cause irregular menstruation. In addition, inflammation and tumor of the reproductive organs and disorder of the endocrine system, mental disorders, constitutional and environmental changes and disorders of other organs may also give rise to the disease.

Essential of Diagnosis

1. Unsmooth discharge of mense, preceded or delayed menstruation, little or great in volume and abnormal mense color, accompanied with lassitude, anemia, dizziness and indigestion.

2. Most patients with their menstruation occurring 10 days earlier than the normal time, being red in color and great in volume, have vexation, red face and a hot sensation; those with their menstruation occurring 10 days later than the normal time, with a dark and scanty mense, usually have general weakness, pale, aversion to cold and desire for warmth; and those with their menstruation occurring at irregular times, either preceded or delayed, have emaciation, dizziness, soreness of loins, dark and grey face, great or less mense which is also light in color, and chest distension.

Massage Treatment

1. Prescription of foot points: Press and knead bilateral Zusanli, Xuehai and Ququan; point and knead bilateral Sanyinjiao, Diji and Ligou; pinch and knead bilateral Taichong, Taixi and Zhaohai; and knead heavily bilateral Gongsun, Shuiquan and Bafeng.

2. Prescription of foot reflecting zones: Push and press Adrenal Gland and Kidney in sequence on the soles of feet; point and knead Pituitary Gland, Thyroid Gland and Genital Gland in the soles; point and knead Celliac Plexus and Liver in the right sole; push and press Heart and Spleen in the left sole; grasp and push Lower Abdomen and Genital Gland in the medial side of the dorsum of feet and Uterus in the lateral side of the dorsum from upper to lower.

Remarks

1. The above point or zone groups are to be treated twice a day. This therapy should be started $5 \sim 7$ days before a menstruation, and is resumed again before next menstruation. Better therapeutic effect can be obtained if this therapy can be applied continuously for several months.

2. Pay attention to menstrual hygiene, eat less cold or raw or irritative food, avoid emotional stimuli and do less physical work.

3. If this disease is caused by tumors, surgical therapy should be employed.

Dysmenorrhea

This refers to the abdominal pain occurring during, before or after the menstruation. If it has occurred in one's first menstruation without notable organic diseases of the reproductive organs, it is known as primary dysmenorrhea; if it is caused by organic diseases of the reproductive organs after the first menstruation, it is a secondary dysmenorrhea. In most cases, dysmenorrhea is caused by maldevelopment of the uterus, incoordinative uterine contraction or excessive uterine contraction which, again, causes ischemia of the uterus and the ensuing pain. It may also be caused by stricture of the cervical neck which gives rise to unsmooth discharge of mense. Dysmenorrhea due to failure of the large patchy endometrium to be discharged through opening of the uterus is called membranous dysmenorrhea. As a result of congestion, bleeding or adhesion due to inflammation of the pelvic cavity or shifting of the endometrium may also lead to dysmenorrhea. In addition, emotional disturbance or constitutional variations are closely related to dysmenorrhea.

Essential of Diagnosis

1. The colicky pain in the lower abdomen usually occurs on the 1st or the 2nd day after a menstruation begins and may radiate to the vagina, anus and loins, companied with breast distending pain in some cases.

2. Patients often have such manifestations as nausea, vomiting, headache or even pale, cold sweating, cold limbs and restlessness.

3. The pain gradually disappears with discharge of mense, but patients with membranous dysmenorrhea often experience severe pain on the 3rd or the 4th day after the menstruation begins, which is relieved after the membranous substance is discharged.

Massage Treatment

1. Prescription of foot points: Press and knead bilateral Zusanli and Xuehai; point and knead bilateral Sanyinjiao and Diji; and knead heavily bilateral Taichong, Gongsun and Taibai.

2. Prescription of foot reflecting zones: Push and press from Kid-

ney to Bladder through Ureter and push and press Genital Gland in the soles; grasp and push Uterus and Vagina in the medial side of the dorsums of the feet; press and knead Genital Gland in the lateral side of the dorsums of feet; push and press Lymph Gland of Upper Body and Lymph Gland of Lower Body from lower to upper; pinch and knead Lymph Gland of the Whole Body toe by toe.

Remarks

1. The above point or zone groups are to be treated twice a day. If rubbing lower abdomen 30~50 times in each treatment is also adopted, the therapeutic effect will be even better.

2. Patients should pay attention to menstrual hygiene and the hygiene of sexual life and avoid emotional stimuli, invasion of cold and over intake of cold or raw food.

3. This disease may be caused by many other diseases. So it is necessary to perform the gynecological examinations in order to make a definite diagnosis. For secondary dysmenorrhea, the primary diseases must be treated.

Amenorrhea

If a female over 18 years old does not experience any menstruation, it is called primary amenorrhea; while if menstruation stops for more than 3 months after the first menstruation, it is called secondary amenorrhea.

Normal menstruation depends on coordinative activities of the hypothalamus-pituitary gland-ovarum axis and the periodiac reactions of the endometrium to the sexual hormone. If organic or functional disturbance happens to any of the above links, amenorrhea will develop.

Essential of Diagnosis

1. Occurrence of the disease is often related to disorders of the endocrine system, emotions and nerve. These factors can be classified as two types, the general type and the local type. The former includes chronic diseases, anemia and malnutrition; while the latter

indicates congenital maldevelopment of the reproductive organs, tuberculosis or tumor of the reproductive organs, and atrophy of uterus. Amenorrhea may also be caused by affection of cold, over fatigue or severe emotional injury during menstruation.

2. Amenorrhea secondary to general disorders is often accompanied with emaciation, dry skin, pale lips, lethargy, occasional low fever, night sweat, dizziness, palpitation, soreness of loins and back, lowering-down pain in the lower abdomen, or dizziness, insomnia, fall of hair, pale, cold sweating, cold limbs or even syncope in severe cases.

3. Amenorrhea due to local disorders is usually associated with distending pain in the lower abdomen, soreness of loins and back, insomnia, restlessness, which are more obvious in adelescent female at the time when the menstruation should have come in a month, and the pain is usually aggravated month by month.

Massage Treatment

1. Prescription of foot points: Press and knead bilateral Zusanli, Xuehai and Ligou; point and knead bilateral Sanyinjiao, Taixi and Fenglong; pinch and knead bilateral Taichong and Gongsun.

2. Press and knead bilateral Pituitary Gland and Genital Gland in the soles; and push and press bilateral Uterus and Vagina on the dorsum of feet.

Remarks

1. The above point or zone groups are to be treated twice a day. If rubbing the lower abdomen 30~50 times in each treatment is also adopted, the therapeutic effect will be even better.

2. This therapy is not effective for the amenorrhea due to congenital abnormality of the reproductive organs.

Breast Distending Pain during Menstruation

This is one of the manifestations of premenstrual tension syndrome which is caused by dysfunction of the subcortical center of the brain and vegetative dysfunction secondary to emotional stress and disorders of sexual hormone secretion.

Essential of Diagnosis

Breast distending pain 3 or 4 days before menstruation or during or after menstruation, with redness and hotness of the breast or even palpable small masses in the breasts. The pain is the most severe in the nipples, which is aggravated by touching, or the nipple is itching and painful with pus discharge, accompanied with distension of the chest and hypochondrium, frequent sighing, or dry eyes, dry mouth and hotness with restlessness which are rapidly relieved after the emenstruation.

Massage Treatment

1. Prescription of the foot points: Press and knead bilateral Zusanli, Fenglong and Xiajuxu; point and knead bilateral Taichong and Xingjian; and pinch and knead bilateral Yongquan.

2. Prescription of the foot reflecting zones: Push and press from Kidney to Bladder through Ureter in the bilateral soles; press and knead Genital Gland in the bilateral soles; push and press bilateral Uterus and Vagina in the medial side of the dorsums of the feet and the Genital Gland in the lateral side of the dorsum of feet; and push and press Thorax on the dorsum of feet from anterior to posterior.

Remarks

1. The above point or zone groups are to be treated twice a day. Usually this therapy should begin $5 \sim 7$ days before menstruation and long-standing application of this therapy has a better therapeutic effect.

2. Keep a calm mind and a pleasant mood and avoid mental stress before menstruation, pay more attention to the daily life and psychologic health during the menstruation.

Abnormal Leukerrhea

Normal leukerrhea is a tasteless thick substance white in color, which comes from mixture of the secretion from the mucous membrane of vagina, glands of the cervex and the endometrium. Abnormality of leukerrhea means increase of the leukerrhea in volume or abnormality of the leukerrhea in quality.

Essential of Diagnosis

1. Simple leukorrhagia: Seen mostly in preovulatory phase, around menstruation, pregnant period or after application of estrin in which the exudate and the secretion increases. This kind of leukorrhea is mucous and tasteless.

2. Purulent leukorrhea: Yellow and mucous leukorrhea with a foul odor is mostly caused by cervical erosin, vaginitis, pelvic inflammation, tumors or infection of the genitals.

3. Bloody leukorrhea: This means that the leukorrhea is stained with blood, which is mostly seen in senile vaginitis, pylop or tumor of the cervix.

4. Bean-curb like or curb mass leukorrhea: This is usually caused by fungal vaginitis.

5. Rice soup leukorrhea with a fishy and fetid odour: This arises from necrosis and degeneration of the advanced cancer tissues of the genital.

6. Most patients has increased viginal secretion, pain in the lower abdomen, soreness of loins, lassitude, dizziness, restlessness and dry mouth.

Massage Treatment

1. Prescriptions of the foot points: Press and knead bilateral Zusanli and Yinlingquan; point and knead bilateral Ligou and Zhaohai; pinch and knead bilateral Sanyinjiao, Taichong, Xingjian, Gongsun and Taibai.

2. Prescription of the foot reflecting zones: Push and press from Adrenal Gland to Bladder through Kidney and Ureter in sequence; push and press Genital Gland; push and press Liver in the right sole from lower to upper and the Spleen in the left sole from the upper to lower; point and knead Celliac Plexus in bilateral soles; push and press Uterus and Vagina in the medial side of the dorsum of feet and Genital Gland in the lateral side of the dorsum; and point and knead Lymph Gland of the Upper Body and the Lymph Gland of the Lower Body on the dorsum of feet.

Remarks

1. The above point or zone groups are to be treated twice a day. If rubbing the lower abdomen clockwise and counterclockwise respectively for 30~50 times in each treatment is also adopted, the therapeutic effect will be even better.

2. This therapy is ineffective for abnormal leukorrhea due to tumors.

Acute Mastitis

This is an acute pyogenic inflammation of the breast caused by invasion of bacteria into the mammary glands or lobules of the mammary gland.

Essential of Diagnosis

1. Seen mostly in lactation of primipara or 3~4 weeks after delivery.

2. Such induction factors as crack, depression or deformity of the nipples, press of the breast or stangnancy of milk in the breast before development of the disease.

3. Initially, the breast is painful and swollen with a red skin. Its local area becomes hard with tenderness. In a few days, the inflammatory mass is softened to be abscess, producing a wave feeling. The auxillary nodes are usually enlarged with tenderness.

4. Such general toxic symptoms as higher fever, chilld, headache, nausea and poor appetite or even septicemia in severe cases present.

Massage Treatment

1. Prescription of foot points: Press and knead bilateral Zusanli, Xiajuxu and Fenglong; point and knead bilateral Sanyinjiao, Taichong, Xingjian and Zulingqi.

2. Prescription of the foot reflecting zones: Point and knead Pituitary Gland in the bilateral soles; push and press continuously from Adrenal Gland to Bladder through Kidney and Ureter and Genital Gland; point and press Spleen in the left sole and Liver in the right

sole; push and press Lymph Gland of the Upper Body, Lymph Gland of the Lower Body, and Lymph Gland of the Chest on the dorsums of feet as well as Genital Gland in the lateral side of the dorsum of feet.

Remarks

1. The above point or zone groups are to be treated twice a day. It will be more effective if gentle massage and kneading on the hard nodules of the breast is adopted at the same time.

2. This therapy has a better therapeutic effect on the early or middle stage of the acute mastitis. Comprehensive measures should be taken for cases with formation of pus or diabrosis or those with general symptoms such as high fever and delirium.

Vomiting of Pregnancy

This disease is a morbid condition marked by severe pregnant reaction with severe vomiting as its main manifestation which often leads to dehydration or acidosis.

Essential of Diagnosis

1. Early pregnancy complicated by frequent vomiting: The vomitus contains not only the food or mucous fluid, but also bile or blood, and patient is unable to eat.

2. Listlessness, lassitude, emaciation and dehydration: In even severe cases, hypotension, fever, rapid pulse or jaundice due to liver injury, or optic neuritis or retinal bleeding in the fundus.

Massage Treatment

1. Prescription of the foot points: Press and knead bilateral Zusanli and Yanglingquan; point and knead bilateral Fenglong and Sanyinjiao; pinch and knead bilateral Taichong and Gongsun.

2. Prescription of the foot reflecting zones: Push and press continuously from Kidney to Bladder through Ureter, Stomach, Duodenum and Genital Gland; push and press Diaphragm on the dorsum of feet from the middle to the lateral sides; grasp and push the Genital Gland in the medial and lateral sides from lower to upper.

Remarks

1. The above points or zone groups are to be treated twice a day. The manipulations applied in the treatment should be gentle and slow and violent or strong stimuli should be avoided.

2. When severe manifestations of dehydration or acidosis occur, combined Chinese and Western measures should be applied.

Prolapse of Uterus

When the uterus goes down from its normal position with the cervix reaching a level below the spine of ischium and the uterus going out of the opening of the vagina, it is known as prolapse of uterus, which is often accompanied with knuckle of the anterior or posterior wall of the vagina. Injury or relaxation of the ligaments, tendons or muscles supporting the uterus or factors that can increase the abdominal pressure can all lead to the disease.

Essential of Diagnosis

It is manifested as a mass that comes out of the vagina, which is small and can retract itself after lying flat in the early stage. In chronic cases, the mass is bigger and is exposed as a result of failure to retract itself. This exposed mass then often develops dryness, fracture, erosion or infection, with a lowering-down sensation, soreness of loins, difficult defecation, retention or incontinence of urine or urinary infection.

Massage Treatment

1. Prescription of foot points: Press and knead bilateral Zusanli and Sanyinjiao; point and knead bilateral Zhaohai and Gongsun; pinch and knead bilateral Shuiquan and Dadun; and rub bilateral Yongquan.

2. Prescription of foot reflecting zones: Push and press Kidney in the soles of feet; point and knead Adrenal Gland; push and press bilateral Uterus and Vagina in the medial sides of the dorsums of feet, Lower Abdomen in the lateral side of the dorsum and Celliac Plexus in the soles of feet.

Remarks
1. The above points or zone groups are to be treated twice a day. The therapeutic effect will be even better if the lower abdomen is also rubbed for 30~50 times and the Baihui point, which is in the center of the vertex, is pressed and kneaded in each of the treatment.
2. Avoid taking part in heavy labor work or standing long and keep defecation smooth to prevent elevation of abdominal pressure.
3. In the treatment, the prolapsed uterus should be pushed above the vagina first and the position of the pelvic cavity raised, and after the treatment patient should keep a chest-knee position for 30 minutes in order to enhance the therapeutic effect.

Postpartum Hypogalactio

This is mostly caused by weak constitution, emotional depression or a low spirit.
Essential of Diagnosis
Inadequate or even no milk is secreted from mammary gland after delivery. The breasts are soft without a distending sensation.
Massage Treatment
1. Prescription of foot points: Press and knead bilateral Zusanli and Ququan; point and knead bilateral Fenglong and Sanyinjiao; and pinch and knead bilateral Taichong, Gongsun and Dadun.
2. Prescription of foot reflecting zones: Press and knead Cerebrum in the bilateral soles; point and knead bilateral Pituitary Gland and Thyroid Gland of the bilateral soles; push and knead bilateral Adrenal Gland and Kidney continuously; point and press Celliac Plexus in the bilateral soles; and push and press Lymph Gland of Upper Body and Thymus Gland on the dorsum of feet.
Remarks
1. The above point or zone groups are to be treated twice a day, and it has a better therapeutic effect on the disease.
2. In the treatment, patient should keep a pleasant mood, have a

proper nutrition, drink more soups, have a good rest and correct the incorrect feeding methods.

Pelvic Inflammation

This disease includes inflammation of the internal genital (uterus, oviduct and ovary), pelvic peritonitis and inflammation of the pelvic connective tissues. It can be classified as the acute and the chronic and it may be either localized or diffusive. In most cases, however, it involves several organs and inflammation of these organs are collectively termed pelvic inflammation in the clinic. Invasion of bacteria in the process of delivery or abortion is the most important cause of the disease, and sexual intercourse during menstruation or spread of appendicitis also serves as the causative factors.

Essential of Diagnosis

1. Acute pelvic inflammation: In the case of acute inflammation of the endometrium, there is elevation of body temperature. acceleration of pulse rate, headache, poor appetite, abdominal distension, uterine pain on touching, increase of vaginal discharge which is purulent in nature or mixed with little blood and foul in smell. When the inflammation spreads to the oviduct and the ovarum, there is pain in one side or bilateral sides of the lower abdomen and continuous elevation of body temperature, and streak-like substance or mass can be clearly palpated beside the uterus. If it is an abscess, undulant mass can be touched. When inflammation happens to the connective tissues and the pelvic perineum simultaneously, there will be sudden elevation of the body temperature, chills, nausea, vomiting, diffusive pain in the lower abdomen which radiates to the thighs bilaterally, accompanied with difficulty in passing urine, frequent urination, a lowering-down sensation during defecation, and sorenss in the back and the lower back.

2. Chronic pelvic inflammation: This condition mostly develops from acute pelvic inflammation that fails to be treated in time or thoroughly. Its main manifestations are: a lowering-down pain in

the lower abdomen which is more severe during menstruation, increased leukorrhea, low fever, lassitude, menorrhagia or prolonged menstrual period. It often present an acute attack after a menstruation. If the oviduct is obstructed due to inflammation, there will be secondary sterility.

Massage Treatment

1. Prescriptions of foot points: Press and knead bilateral Yinlingquan and Sanyinjiao; point and knead bilateral Ligou and Diji; pinch and press bilateral Taichong and Gongsun; and rub bilateral Yongquan.

2. Prescription of foot reflecting zones: Push and press from Adrenal Gland to Bladder through Kidney and Ureter of the soles; press and knead Accessory Thyroid Gland and Genital Gland in the soles; press and knead Spleen in the left sole and Liver in the right sole at fixed points; push and press Lympatic Gland of the Lower Body in the bilateral soles; Uterus in the medial side of the dorsum of feet and the Lower Abdomen and Genital Gland in the lateral side of the dorsum of feet.

Remarks

1. The above point or zone groups are to be treated twice a day. If rubbing lower abdomen clockwise and counterclockwise for 30~50 times is also adopted, better therapeutic effects can be obtained.

2. This disease is caused by a number of factors, so gynecological examinations should be carried out to make a definite diagnosis. If necessary, combined Chinese and Western medicines should be given.

Diseases of the Mouth, Ears, Eyes and Nose

Toothache

This is a most commonly seen symptom in mouth diseases. It may be caused by caries, pericoronitis, acute or chronic pancreatitis, trigerminal neuralgia, etc. Caries is the most frequently encountered mouth disease, which causes toothache as a result of attachment of bacteria to the teeth surface, destruction of hard tissues of the teeth and the ensuing defect of the tooth body.

Essential of Diagnosis

1. If patient has a caries which causes tooth cavities of varying depths, the destruction will be limited to the tooth surface and thus there is not any subjective symptoms. When the disease involves the deeper layer, there will be an increased sensitivity to cold, heat, acid or sweat. When the caries destruction is close to the tooth marrow, there will be severe pain in case of either exposure to cold or heat or remaining of food in the tooth cavity. The pain will be relieved at once when the stimuli is removed.

2. If the diseases penetrates the tooth marrow cavity, inflammation of the tooth marrow will follow. In this case, there will be spontaneously severe toothache which occurs intermittently although there is not external stimuli. At the later stage of inflammation of tooth marrow, the interval between two attacks is shortened. Most patients experience aggravated toothache at night or in a lying position. At the early stage, variations of temperature can aggravate the toothache; while in the advanced stage, the pain is extremely sensitive to heat. Pain in pyogenic flammation of the tooth marrow can be alleviated by cold.

Massage Treatment

1. Prescription of foot points: Press and knead bilateral Zusanli and Sanyinjiao; point and knead bilateral Neiting, Taixi, tip of the medial malleolus and the external malleolus; and pinch and press Bafeng, Niuxi and Lidui.

2. Prescription of foot reflecting zones: Push and press Stomach, Duodenum, Small Intestine and Large Intestine in the bilateral soles; push and press continuously from Kidney to Bladder through Ureter in the soles; and push and knead Upper Palate and Lower Palate on the dorsums of feet.

Remarks

1. The above point or zone groups are to be treated twice a day and this therapy is very effective for the disease.

2. If it is caused by caries, inflammation of the bone marrow or osteomyelitis of jaw, comprehensive therapeutic measures should be taken.

Chronic Rhinitis

This is a commonly seen chronic inflammation of the nasal mucosa and the submucous layer of the nose, which is clinically divided into two types, the chronic simple rhinitis and the chronic atrophic rhinitis.

Essential of Diagnosis

1. Chronic simple rhinitis: A history of repeated attacks of acute rhinitis, manifested as intermittent or alternative nasal obstruction which is more severe in a lying position. As there is dilation of blood vessels and increase of gland secretion in nasal mucosa, there is much mucous nasal discharge. Besides, there is chronic congestion and swelling of the nasal mucosa with a smooth surface which is also soft and elastic.

2. Chronic atrophic rhinitis: This is a condition developing from long-standing simple rhinitis. As the tissues of the nasal mucosa have proliferations, the nasal septum is thickened and thus persistent nasal obstruction with difficult mucous or purulent nasal discharge occurs. In addition, there is tinnitus and decline of auditory ability. In the case of long-standing respiration with the mouth opened and stimuli of the secretion, chronic pharygnitis or laryngitis is often present.

Massage Treatment

1. Prescription of foot points: Press and knead bilateral Weizhong and Feiyang; point and knead bilateral Zhaohai, Kunlun and Tonggu; pinch and knead bilateral Nuxi, Lidui and Zhiyin.

2. Prescription of the foot reflecting zones: Point and knead Nose, Frontal Sinus and Accessory Thyroid Gland in the soles;

push and press Lung laterally; press and knead Lymph Gland of the Upper Body on the dorsums of feet at fixed points.
Remarks
1. The above point or zone groups are to be treated twice a day. The therapeutic effect will be even better if the Yingxiang point beside the nares are rubbed, pressed and kneaded at the same time.

2. Patient should keep himself or herself warm to prevent from catching cold. If nasal discharge is frequently mixed with blood and an unpleasant smell, tumor should be considered.

Chronic Pharyngitis

This is a chronic diffusive inflammation of the mucosa and submucous layer of the pharynx and the lymphatic tissues, which is often a part of the chronic inflammation of the upper respiratory tract.
Essential of Diagnosis
This disease is marked by discomfort in the throat, a feeling of foreign body obstructing in the throat, itching, dryness and mild pain of the throat, etc. In some cases, cough and vomiting may also present as a result of stimuli of the secretions. The duration is long and the symptoms of the diseases are intractable and hard to be relieved.
Massage Treatment
1. Prescription of foot points: Press and knead bilateral Weizhong, Yangfu and Yangjiao; point and knead bilateral Taixi, Zhaohai and Rangu; pinch and knead Neiting, Medial Malleolus, Dazhong and Lidui; and pinch, press and rub bilateral Yongquan.

2. Prescription of the foot reflecting zones: Pinch and press with strong force Tonsil, Throat, Trachea, and Lymph Gland of Chest at fixed points; and push and press from upper to lower the Lymph Gland of the Upper Body, the Lymph Gland of the Lower Body and the Lymph Gland of the Whole Body in the bilateral sides of the ankle.
Remarks

1. Long-standing application of this therapy by massaging the above point or zone groups twice a day has a remarkable effect on the chronic laryngitis.

2. During the treatment, patient should keep away from smoking and alcohol and has a food containing less oil or fat, and after eating, in the morning or in the evening, he or she should rinse his or her mouth.

3. If an aged patient experiences aggravated hoarseness which fails to be cured in a long time, the possibility of tumor should be considered.

Tonsilitis

This is a kind of infection of the lymphatic tissues in the larynx, which is the most severe in tonsils. It has two types, the acute tonsilitis and the chronic tonsilitis, which are both caused by streptococcus B. In a healthy person, the bacteria exist in the larynx and the tonsilar crypts, which will induce the disease when the resistant ability of the body is lowered.

Essential of Diagnosis

1. Acute tonsilitis: Seen mostly in children or young people. According to its clinical features, it can be classified as three types: the acute catarrhal tonsilitis, the acute cryptsal tonsilitis and the acute follicular tonsilitis. The acute catarrhal tonsilitis is mild in condition and is marked by fever, sore throat, and congestion and swelling of the tonsil and mucous membrane of the palate arc; the acute cryptsal tonsilitis has a sudden onset with severe local and general manifestations such as marked sore throat and pain in swallowing which may radiate to the ear region, fever, enlarged tonsil and spot secretion yellow-white in color in the crypts or pseudo-membrane in the crypts; and the acute follicular tonsilitis is also sudden in onset with more severe local and general symptoms such as high fever, chills, convulsion and vomiting in children, obviously enlarged and congested tonsil, in the submucosal layer between the crypts, yellow-

white small prominence formed by pus. In addition, patient may have enlarged lymph nodes in the region below the mandibles, which are painful on pressing.

2. Chronic tonsilitis: There is a history of repeated attack of the acute tonsilitis. At the remission stage, it may be asymptomatic. Patient may have chronic congestion of the tonsils and the palatoglossal arc and scar or yellow-white spots in the surface of the tonsils. In children, there may be hyperplasia of the tonsil which will influence respiration and swallowing. If it is complicated by adenoid enlargement, it may cause nasal obstruction, snoring during sleep and enlargement of the lymph nodes below the mandibles.

Massage Treatment

1. Prescription of foot points: Press and knead bilateral Weizhong and Yangjiao; point and press bilateral Zhaohai and Taixi; pinch and knead bilateral Neiting, Rangu, Tip of the Medial Malleolus and Lidui.

2. Prescription of the foot reflecting zones: Press and knead Tonsil, Lower Palate, Lymph Gland of the Upper Body, Lymph Gland of the Chest and Lymph Gland of the Whole Body on the dorsums of feet; press and knead toe by toe Frontal Sinus in the soles; and press and push Spleen in the left sole.

Remarks

1. The above point or zone groups are to be treated twice a day. The manipulations for the acute tonsilitis should be a little heavy so that the pain can be relieved quickly. For the chronic cases, the manipulation should be gentle and slow and lasts a longer time. Constant application of this therapy has a better therapeutic effect for the disease. If pressing and kneading the painful point below the manidibles is also adopted, the effect will be even better.

2. Patient should keep him or her warm, prevent himself or herself from being caught by cold, eat less acrid and pungent food; and avoid smoking or drinking.

Otitis Media Suppurativa

This is a diseases caused by invasion of purulent bacteria into the ear through otosalpinx, traumatically injured drum membrane or blood stream, mostly secondary to acute infection of the upper respiratory tract. Clinically, it can be divided into two types, the acute and the chronic. The chronic type is often secondary to an acute one due to delayed or incomplete treatment.

Essential of Diagnosis

1. Acute otitis media suppurativa: The ear pain is aggravated progressively, being throbbing pain in nature, which may influence sleep in severe cases. When perforation of the drum membrane occurs, the pain will be relieved remarkably at once. There may be sound conduction deafness which is accompanied with deafness. The general manifestations include fever, chills, headache and general discomfort.

2. Chronic otitis media suppurativa: This disease is mainly characterized by long-standing or intermittent pus discharge, perforation of drum membrane and deafness. It has three types: ① Simple type, which is marked by intermittent or persistent discharge of mucous pus which is not fetid in odor and extensive central perforation of the drum membrane; ② Caries type, which is marked by persistent pus discharge with a foul smell and large or boundary perforation of the drum membrane; ③ The third type, which is marked by peristent discharge of foul and fishy pus, and boundary perforation of perforation in the relaxant zone, accompanied with tinnitus and dizziness in some cases.

Massage Treatment

1. Prescription of the foot points: Press and knead bilateral Yanglingquan and Fenglong; point and knead bilateral Zhaohai, Taixi and Neiting; pinch and knead Bilateral Xiaxi, Zulinqi and Jinmen; and knead with more strength and rub bilateral Yongquan.

2. Prescription of foot reflecting zones: Press and knead at a fixed point Accessory Thyroid Gland, Ear, Trigerminal Nerve and

Frontal Sinus; push and press constantly from Kindey to Bladder through Ureter; push and press Lymph Gland of the Upper Body, Lymph Gland of the Lower Body, Lymph Gland of the Chest and the Labyrinth.

Remarks
1. The above point or zone groups, to be treated twice a day, have some effects on the disease.

2. When there is exudation of pus from the auditory tract, external therapy should be applied jointly to clean the auditory tract. If perforation happens to the drum membrane, application of this therapy alone is not effective, and special treatment should be taken.

3. Patient should avoid eating acrid, pungent, dry-hot or fishy food, and less fatty or greasy food is recommended.

Motorcycle and Boat Sickness

This is a kind of clinical manifestation marked by simultaneous changes of the gastrointestinal tract, inner ear and the heart.

Essential of Diagnosis
Being shaked by motion of motorcycle or boat for a long time, the human body will produce dizziness due to functional disturbance of the balance organs of the inner ear. The external stimuli is transmitted to the sympathetic nerve, causing tachycardia and disturbance of the gastrointestinal tract. Elevation of the abdominal pressure will give rise to upward flow of the gastric contents, leading to nausea and vomiting. Besides, some people may experience dizziness, vomiting and palpitation because they are very sensitive to the odor of the gas or oil discharged by the motorcycle or boat or due to sound interferance, and some people may feel dizzy on taking on the motorcycle or boat as a result of their terror or nervous excessive sensitivity.

Massage Treatment
1. Prescription of foot points: Press and knead bilateral Zusanli,

Fenglong and Sanyinjiao; point and knead bilateral Jiexi, Taixi and Taichong; and pinch and knead bilateral Zhiyin and Yonquan.

2. Prescription of foot reflecting zones: Push and press Cerebellum, Trigerminal Nerve, Temporal Lobe, Ear and Celliac Plexus; push and press bilateral Stomach, Pancreas and Duodenum in the soles; push and press Heart in the left sole from lower to upper; and push and press Labyrinth on the dorsum of feet forward to the tips of toes.

Remarks

1. The above point or zone groups are to be treated twice a day. Long-term application of this therapy can relieve the response of the motorcycle or boat sickness.

2. Patient should calm his or her mind when he or she takes motorcycle or boat. Be sure not to be nervous. If this therapy is also adopted simultaneously, better therapeutic effect can be obtained.

Myopia

Myopia refers to a morbid state of the eye marked by the focus of a parallel light reflected by the eye being anterior to the retina in the case of the eye pressure requiring no adjustment. It is often caused by a longer anterio-posterior axis or a strong refraction force of the eyeball.

Essential of Diagnosis

1. Failure to see far objects clearly or decline of the ability to see far and a normal ability to see objects in a short distance. The near point in severe myopia may shift to just anterior to the ear.

2. The anterio-posterior axis, especially the posterior part of the eyeball is prolonged, with mild prominence of the eyeball in severe cases. It is usually progressive and is related to hereditary factors.

3. In severe myopia, there are turbidity and liquecation of the vetrieous body and the changes of fundus in myopia. When retinal tear occurs, retinal detachment often follows.

4. Extrotropia may present as a result of weakening of conver-

gence.
Massage Treatment
1. Prescription of foot points: Press and knead bilateral Zusanli and Sanyinjiao; point and knead bilateral Guangming, Taichong and Zhaohai; pinch and knead bilateral Rangu, Zulinqi and Xiaxi.

2. Prescription of foot reflecting zones: Push and press from Kidney to Bladder through Ureter in the soles; push and knead Frontal Sinus toe by toe; point and press Eyes and Genital Glands in the soles and the Liver in the right sole; and push and press Uterus in the medial side of the dorsums of feet and the Genital Gland in the lateral side of the dorsum of feet.

Remarks
1. The above point or zone groups are to be treated twice a day. If this treatment is used together with the massage at the points around the eyes with an aim to keeping health in adolescent myopia, the effects will be even better.

2. Patients should correct their unfavorable habits in reading, improve their constitutions and protect their eyes while receiving the treatment.

3. This therapy is not effective for myopia caused by congenital defect or maldevelopment of the eyeball.

Aphtha

This disease is the most commonly seen damage in membranous diseases of the oral cavity, which is characterized by its periodiac attacks, so it is also called repeated aphtha.

Essential of Diagnosis
1. This disease tends to occur in the zone where the stratum corneum is poor, such as the inner side of the lips, the tongue tip or the soft palate.

2. The erosion is usually single round or an oval lesion superficially seated, $2\sim3$mm in diameter with a red and swollen border. Its center is a little yellow and depressed and it gives rise to a bur-

ning pain. Mostly, the disease will heal in 7~10 days, but it tends to attack periodically and influence appetite.

Massage Treatment

1. Prescription of foot points: Press and knead bilateral Zusanli and Sanyinjiao; point and knead bilateral Zhaohai, Neiting and Gongsun; pinch and knead bilateral Lidui; and pinch, knead and rub bilateral Yongquan.

2. Prescription of foot reflecting zones: Hold and twist Frontal Sinus of soles toe by toe; push and press Stomach, Duodenum and Small Intestine in the soles, Spleen in the left sole and Gallbladder and Liver in the right sole; push and press from Kidney to Bladder through Ureter.

Remarks

1. The above points or zone groups are to be treated twice a day. Constant application of this therapy has a better therapeutic effect on the disease.

2. Massage on the adjacent zones of the aphtha should be adopted simultaneously in order to gain even better therapeutic effect. The procedures of the massage are: Wash the hands clean first, then make the thumb and the index finger face each other, and put one finger into the oral cavity to touch the zone around the aphtha and put the other finger in a corresponding position out of the mouth. After that, knead and pinch the gently and softly for about 10 seconds. This procedure is to be repeated in 3~4 points around the aphtha.

3. Patients should have a regular daily life and enough sleep, avoid eating much pungent, acrid or irritative food, eat more vegetables and fruits, and keep their defecation smooth.

Presbytia

When seeing near in a healthy condition, the ciliary muscle will contract, the suspensorium will become relaxant, and the anterior surface of the crystalloid body will be depressed. As a result, increase of the **refractive power leads** to the focus staying in the retina, which is known as adjustment. In the middle-aged or the aged people, however, the core of the crystalloid body becomes hard gradually and its adjustment ability is lowered with increase of age. So, difficulty in reading or work by seeing near is referred to as presbytia, occurs.

Essential of Diagnosis

1. Patient has a normal far vision but a poor near vision. When he or she reads or works, he or she has to move away from the objects for some distance in order to see clearly, and if the reading or seeing lasts some time, he or she will present the symptoms of eye fatigue.

2. In severe cases of presbytia, patients will still fail to see clearly even the near point is drawing far.

Massage Treatment

1. Prescription of foot points: Press and knead bilateral Zusanli, Yanglingquan and Sanyinjiao; point and knead bilateral Guangming and Taichong; pinch and knead bilateral Shuiquan and Zulinqi; and rub bilateral Yongquan.

2. Prescription of foot reflecting zones: Pinch and knead Frontal Sinus toe by toe; press Eyes in the soles at fixed points; push and press from Kidney to Bladder through Ureter.

Remarks

1. The above point or zone groups are to be treated twice a day. Constant application of this therapy has a better therapeutic effect in protecting vision in middle-aged or senile patients.

2. If warming-eye therapy is adopted jointly, the therapeutic effect will be even better. The warming-eye therapy is performed as follows: First rub the palms of hands until a hot sensation is produced, then apply the center of the palms on the eyeballs and knead the eye gently and slowly for 1～2 minutes.

Dermatological Diseases

Common Comedo

This is an inflammation caused by hypersteatosis following maturity of the sebaceous gland and kerotoma of the epithelium of the follicular orifice which obstructs in the opening of the sebaceous gland and causes the secondary bacterial infection.

Essential of Diagnosis

1. Seen mostly in adolescent people and in the face or chest.

2. Initially, it presents as small eruption with a normal skin color, then, it turns gradually from yellow to dark. When the black tip is removed, there is a cylinder-like substance, which is known as comedo with a black tip. In addition, it may also occur as the comedo of pustule type, hard nodular type or the cystoma type.

3. It is a chronic disease which may heal itself after 30 years old.

4. If no infection occurs, no subjective symptoms will be exhibited.

Massage Treatment

1. Prescription of foot points: Press and knead bilateral Zusanli and Xiajuxu; point and knead bilateral Sanyinjiao, Neiting and Weizhong; and pinch and knead bilateral Taichong, Zuqiaoyin and Yongquan.

2. Prescription of foot reflecting zones: Push and press from Adrenal Gland to Bladder through Kidney and Ureter and the Genital Gland in the soles; point and knead Pituitary Gland in the soles; push and press Lung and Trachea; Push and knead in the direction of intestines Large Intestine in bilateral soles, the Liver, the Gallbladder in the right sole and the Genital Gland in the medial and lateral sides of the dorsum of feet.

Remarks

1. The above point or zone groups are to be treated twice a day.

2. Patient should avoid eating much acrid, pungent, fatty and greasy food. Smoking and drinking are forbidden, and he or she

should eat more vegetable or fruits.

Eczema

This is an allergic skin disorder caused by multiple internal or external factors acting on a specific body. It is marked by multiple skin lesions and is divided into three types, the acute, the subacute and the chronic.

Essential of Diagnosis
1. Acute eczema: The skin lesions are multiple in shapes, presenting as edemous erythoma, blister, erosion with exudation, scar formation or even infection. Mostly, 2 or 3 of the above skin lesions are dominant, which have a poorly defined border. If it is seen in the head or face and the flexor side of the limbs, it is usually symmetrical. And, it often gives rise to severe pain and lasts $2 \sim 3$ weeks. It has a tendency of relapse.

2. Subacute eczema: This condition mostly arises from acute one, which has a slow progress with mild inflammation and less exudation. Small amount of dequamation or scar may be noted.

3. Chronic eczema: It is often primary or develops from subacute eczema, mostly appearing in the retroauditory region, scrotum or the lower leg. In the affected zone, there are roughening and thickening of skin, deep skin wrinkles, pigmentation, scractching edge and dequamation. In the case of keratosis occurs, cracks will appear. In addition, this condition often presents itching.

Massage Treatment
1. Prescription of foot point: Press and knead bilateral Weizhong and Yingu; point and knead bilateral Xuehai and Sanyinjiao; and pinch and knead bilateral Dadun.

2. Prescription of foot reflecting zones: Push and press from Adrenal Gland to Bladder through Kidney and Ureter; point and knead Accessory Thyroid Gland; push and press Lung, Trachea and Pituitary Gland; press and knead Spleen in the left sole at a fixed point; push and knead Large Intestine; and push and press Lymph

Gland of the Upper Body, Lymph Gland of the Lower Body and Lymph Gland of the Chest on the dorsums of feet.

Remarks

1. The above point or zone groups are to be treated twice a day, and this therapy has a better therapeutic effect on the disease.

2. Try best to find out the causative factors of the disease so that the treatment can be conducted directing at the causes.

Urticaria

This is an allergic disease marked by skin papulas caused by some factors.

Essential of Diagnosis

1. The skin lesions are manifested as papulas of varying sizes, light red or normal in color, which appear and disappear rapidly. It may appear several times a day.

2. The acute urticaria may recover in 1~2 weeks. If it lasts more than 6 months, it will become a chronic one.

3. It has such symptoms as itching or chest stuffiness, abdominal pain and diarrhea in some cases.

4. This disease may be only a sign of some diseases. In the acute case, patients often have a history of intake of food containing heteroprotein or drugs, while in the chronic case, chronic diseases or parasitosis are often detected.

Massage Treatment

1. Prescription of foot points: Press and knead bilateral Xuehai, Weizhong and Zusanli; point and knead bilateral Sanyinjiao and Fenglong; and pinch and knead bilateral Neiting and Dadun.

2. Prescription of foot reflecting zones: Push and press from Kidney to Bladder through Ureter; point and knead Pituitary Gland, Thyroid Gland and Accessory Thyroid Gland; point and knead Spleen; push and press Stomach and Duodenum in the soles of the feet.

Remarks

1. The above point or zone groups are to be treated twice a day. This therapy has a better therapeutic effect on the disease. If there is intolerable itching, press and knead Dazhui (in the depression below the spinous process of the 7th cervical vertebra) additionally.

2. The causative factors for chronic urticaria should be found out so that proper measures can be taken.

Neurodermatitis

This is a skin neurosism marked by itching, which is often induced by emotional changes and local fracture. The skin lesion is lichenoid.

Essential of Diagnosis
1. Itching in a local zone, then round or multiple angle skin eraptions, which coalesces into groups, are formed as a result of scratching. In chronic case, the skin folds are deepened and the dermal ridges are prominent, causing the skin to be thickened with a brown color and the ensuing lichenoid changes.

2. This condition can be divided into the localized type and the disseminated type. The former, which is more frequently seen, often appears in the side or back of neck, the flexor or extensor side of the elbow, the medial side of the sacrum or the thigh and the fibular side of the lower leg, while the latter is mainly seen in the face, scapular skin, shoulder, lumbar region, etc.

3. This disease often experiences a chronic course and presents paroxysmal itching.

Massage Treatment
1. Prescription of the foot points: Press and knead bilateral Weizhong and Zusanli; point and knead bilateral Xuehai and Sanyinjiao; and pinch and knead bilateral Neiting, Taichong and Dadun.

2. Prescription of foot reflecting zones: Point and press Cerebrum, Pituitary Gland and Adrenal Gland in the soles; push and press Lung, Trachea and Large Intestine in the bilateral soles; push and press Liver in the right sole and the Heart in the left sole.

Remarks

1. The above point or zone groups are to be treated twice a day. Constant application of this therapy has some effects on the disease.

2. It is generally believed that this disease is related to psychoneurotic factors. If the prescription for neurosism is also adopted, the therapeutic effects will be even better.

Alopecia Areata

This refers to patchy fall of hair in a localized zone, which may be related to emotional changes.

Essential of Diagnosis

1. Sudden occurrence of single or multiple round zone where no hair covers in the head while the skin is normal. If the hair falls completely, it is called complete alopecia, and if all the hairs including the vellus fall, it is termed general alopecia.

2. Seen mostly in the young or children, and in most cases, there is no subjective symptoms.

3. This disease takes a slow course, varying from several months or several years. After that, vellus begins to grow gradually and changes from yellow to black in color and from fine to thick in size.

Massage Treatment

1. Prescription of foot points: Press and knead bilateral Xuehai and Zusanli; point and knead bilateral Sanyinjiao, Taichong and Taixi; pinch and press bilateral Dadun; and rub bilateral Yingquan.

2. Prescription of foot reflecting zones: Twist and knead Frontal Sinus toe by toe; point and knead Cerebrum, Cerebellum, Pituiatry Gland and Trigerminal Nerve in the soles; and push and press from Kidney to Bladder through Ureter.

Remarks

1. The above point or zone groups are to be treated twice a day. Meanwhile, Baihui, which is in the vertex of head, is pressed and kneaded 30~50 times. In addition, fresh ginger should be smeared on the affected zone. Combined use of the above therapies may bring

about remarkable effects.

2. Patients should keep their mind calm and pleasant, take mutiple food and have sufficient sleep. They should avoid washing their hair with strong irritative soap.

Massage on the foot points and the reflecting zones is an important component part of traditional Chinese medicine. It is being more and more widely accepted and its content is becoming more and more plentiful. Treatment of diseases with massage on the points in the feet and reflecting zones in the feet introduced in this book are the general conventional prescriptions. When diseases are to be treated, one should apply these prescriptions flexibly with proper modifications according to changes of illness conditions on the basis of syndromes identified in order to achieve better therapeutic effects. Take viral hepatitis as an example, the points from the liver channels and the Liver and Gallbladder zone in the soles should be specially treated so as to clear away heat and remove Dampness from the liver and gallbladder and restore the normal functions of the liver. Meanwhile, Spleen, Lymph Gland of the Upper Body, Lymph Gland of the Lower Body, Lymph Gland of the Chest and the Liver Meridian Gland should also be adopted as supplementary measures so as to enhance the immunological function of the human body and help the self-recovering ability of the body to give its effect. In addition, the reflecting zones of the Kidney, the Ureter and the Bladder are also treated so that the toxic metabolic products in the human body can be discharged in time.

足部穴区按摩疗法

编　著　单仁颖　于蒙爱
审　校　王国才
翻　译　路玉滨　王　岩
　　　　马欣媛
责任编辑　马万年

*

山东科学技术出版社出版
济南市玉函路 16 号　邮政编码　250002
山东滨州新华印刷厂印刷
中国国际图书贸易总公司发行
中国北京车公庄西路 35 号
北京邮政信箱第 399 号　邮政编码　100044

*

1997 年(大 32 开)　1 版 1 次
ISBN 7—5331—1891—X
R・549
07200
14—E—3027P